Miracle Metabolism

Your Step-by-Step Guide to Quickly Lose Fat, Gain Muscle, and Heal at Any Age

D0905797

Miracle Metabolism

Your Step-by-Step Guide to Quickly Lose Fat, Gain Muscle, and Heal at Any Age

Thomas Tadlock, MS

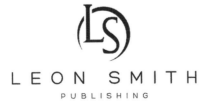

LEON SMITH
PUBLISHING

www.LeonSmithPublishing.com

Dedication

This book is dedicated to my soul mate and the love of my life, my wife. Brooke, it has been through our greatest pains that we have been able to create our greatest gift. We were meant to come together, and it has become our duty to share our amazing, life-altering gift. I love you with everything I am. You are my everything.

Acknowledgments

This book has been wanting to come out of me for a long time. If it weren't for Keith and Maura Leon from the YouSpeakIt Books Program, this book would not exist today. A long time ago, I met Keith Leon, and I told him that I wanted to change the world.

He said, "You've got a book in you, and it needs to come out."

The experience of writing this book has been one that I will forever be grateful for.

Thank you to my wife, my soul mate, my best friend, the one I adore the most, the one I couldn't live without, and who inspired the creation of this book. I love you.

Thank you to all my clients whose dedication to my programs created the basis behind all the principles presented in this book.

Finally, thank you to all my fans. I wrote this for you. Now read it and go make the world a healthier place.

Contents

Introduction   11

CHAPTER ONE
What Is Metabolism, And Is Mine Slow?   19
   Why Metabolism Is Everything
     In Health And Fitness   19
   Self-Test Evaluation: Do You Have A Slow
     Metabolism? Let's Find Out   31
   Let's Start Raising Your Metabolism Today   41

CHAPTER TWO
The Metabolic Miracle — Healing From Disease   65
   The Top *Healthy* Foods
     That Are Hurting Your Health   65
   Curing An Incurable Disease —
     Brooke's Story   72
   How To Heal With Supermarket Foods   81

CHAPTER THREE
Fat Loss Made Fast And Easy   91
   Fat-Loss Nutrition   91
   Fat-Loss Exercise   99
   Putting It Into Practice   132

CHAPTER FOUR

    Building Muscle Quickly At Any Age   153

        Muscle-Building Nutrition   153

        Muscle-Building Exercise   163

        Putting It Into Practice   173

CHAPTER FIVE

    Having It All And Keeping It Forever   195

        The Inconvenient Truths About Fat Loss

          And Muscle Building   195

        Creating Your Dream Body Blueprint   200

        Metabolic Ninja Tactics   208

Conclusion   213

Next Steps   217

About the Author   219

Introduction

What you are about to read—or experience, if you decide to take action on everything that I teach you—will absolutely change your life.

It has changed my life, my family members' lives, and the lives of thousands of my students all over the world. You will learn how to transform your body, with the greatest amount of ease and enjoyment, in a way that will leave you healthier, more energetic, stronger, and fitter. And you'll be able to achieve results quickly, regardless of your age. The information I'm going to share with you is easy to understand, easy to implement, and should make a whole lot of sense.

If you've ever been confused by different fitness information, how to build muscle, how to get lean, and how to raise your metabolism, I've got good news for you—you've picked up the right book.

I am going to help you:

- Understand how to create a healthy body that resists and reverses disease
- Lose all the fat you want
- Gain all the muscle you want
- Maintain it easily, with the least amount of effort

This is true even if you are in your fifties, sixties, or seventies — even your eighties. After reading this book, you will have such a solid understanding of metabolism that you will be able to create and keep any body that you want at any age.

My reason for writing this book is because a long time ago, I was in the worst health of my life. After seeing my best friend die of cancer at twenty-four years old, I took a good look at myself and realized I wasn't very far behind him. As a former computer scientist, I used to spend up to eighty hours a week sitting in front of a computer. My diet consisted mostly of cafeteria food, gummy bears, and personal-size pizzas.

The habits I developed from being overworked, overstressed, and not treating my body well resulted in:

- Hypertension
- High cholesterol
- Clinical depression
- Tendonitis in both shoulders
- Chondromalacia in both knees
- Lower back pain
- Carpal tunnel syndrome in both arms

And I was only twenty-one years old.

I realized I needed to make a big change in my life, so I sought the best information I could possibly find. With that information, I was able to completely transform my body.

With proper exercise and nutrition, I was able to:

- Recover from my depression
- Reverse my hypertension
- Normalize my cholesterol
- Heal my tendonitis
- Heal my chondromalacia
- Eliminate my back pain
- Eliminate my carpal tunnel syndrome
- Sculpt a rock-solid body

This information transformed my life. I starred on MTV and was on the front cover of a fitness magazine.

Since then, I've helped countless others do the same thing. It is so easy and achievable when you know what you're doing and you know the right ways to create the results you want.

I thought: *If a former computer programmer can figure out how to get the health and body of his dreams, then anybody can.*

I feel that I have a duty to get this information to as many people as possible, because it has transformed my body and my life, and it has helped save countless lives.

I have created this book to help you get the body you want. I want to help you become so healthy that you'll be able to live a long, happy life and positively influence all the people whom you love and care for.

I have invested tens of thousands of dollars in my education. What has been so frustrating is that I would apply the things I learned from everything that I was taught, but I would only get results for half the people I worked with. It didn't make sense to me that everybody didn't get the same results, if I was applying the same strategies and skills. I've made it my mission to figure out the real truth.

How do I get results for *everybody*?

What is the key?

What are the missing ingredients I had not been taught in all my certifications and graduate studies on how to transform people's fitness and bodies?

I have found what those ingredients are, and I want to let the world know, so everyone can finally end the struggle of getting fit and getting healthy.

In school, I studied computer science and mathematics. When I graduated, I thought my career path was going to be in software design. I thought that I was going to be a programmer and software developer for the rest of my life.

Every time I teach this information that you're about to learn — whenever I give a talk, hold a webinar, create a program, and now, with my first book on the topic — it creates such a feeling of purpose and satisfaction in me because I know that once you take action, your life is no longer going to be the same.

To get the most out of this book, I recommend you start from the first page and read it all the way through in sequence. Every chapter builds on the previous one, so if you skip ahead, you may miss important ideas and concepts from earlier chapters. I think you will get everything you possibly can out of this book, in the most efficient way possible, by reading the book in the order in which it was written.

When you have finished reading, you will understand metabolism in such a deep way that you'll be able to raise your metabolism — no matter how old you are — and maintain a fast metabolism for the rest of your life.

By implementing the strategies I teach, you will be able to achieve a stronger, leaner, healthier body easily at any age. You will also be able to help your family and friends achieve healthier results.

Let's get started!

CHAPTER ONE

What Is Metabolism, and Is Mine Slow?

WHY METABOLISM IS EVERYTHING IN HEALTH AND FITNESS

Before I was a fitness trainer, I was a computer programmer. I saw everything in my world in terms of algorithms and systems. Once a computer algorithm was in place, it would return the right result every single time.

After I became a fitness trainer, I thought human biology should be no different than a computer program in losing fat and gaining muscle. If I run a weight loss program on my client, they should lose weight. If I run the muscle-building program, their body should gain muscle. The results were sometimes frustratingly unpredictable.

Often clients would lose weight, but some clients would *gain* weight or wouldn't lose any weight at all. This didn't fit into my model of how the world was supposed to work. A program is supposed to work the same way every time — that's what I learned in computer science. When I started understanding biology, I believed that from our lowest level we are all exactly the same.

I wanted to figure out why I was getting these different results with my clients. I wanted to end the frustration for people who couldn't seem to achieve the results they expected.

They wanted to:

- Lose weight
- Build muscle
- Get healthier
- Increase endurance
- Gain strength

I wanted to help everyone who struggled and couldn't seem to make those results occur. That's when I discovered the answer: *metabolism.*

At the lowest level of a computer, programming is nothing more than a set of transistors being operated by ones and zeros. I believed that at the lowest level of our bodies, we are nothing more than cells being operated by molecules. In the world of computer science, if your program returns the wrong result that means you made a mistake in your programming. It's never a problem with the hardware. Once you fix the programming, the computer returns the right results every time.

The reason I wasn't getting the results I wanted with some of my clients was that I didn't quite understand the programming of the human body. Your metabolism is the program your body is currently running.

You can thank your metabolism for:

- How quickly you lose weight
- How much weight you lose
- Your ability to build muscle
- How much muscle you can build
- How quickly you can build muscle
- How healthy you can be
- Your resistance to disease
- How quickly you can recover from disease

Metabolism is everything!

Let me repeat that: it's *everything*.

We'll dive a little deeper into the actual definition, but after working with some of the greatest experts in the world, earning a master's degree and more than eight different national fitness certifications, I have discovered that it is all about metabolism. When I focused on my clients' metabolisms, they all got the right results. And I can't wait to share it with you!

The Biological (Real) Definition of Metabolism

Let's start with what metabolism truly is, because it's probably not what you have been taught. I remember when I learned about metabolism. I was given a definition that was something along the lines of how many calories you're able to burn when you're at rest and how quickly you're able to lose weight. That's how I interpreted the definition of metabolism for many years.

I thought that people with fast metabolisms could lose weight — and lose weight easily. I thought it was merely about weight loss and being able to eat a lot of calories and not have anything noticeable happen to your body. And I thought that for everybody else with a slow metabolism, it wouldn't take much food before they became overweight, and they had to watch everything they ate.

When I did my own research on biology in medical texts, however, I found that that's only part of the definition.

According to Merriam-Webster, the biological definition of metabolism is "the chemical changes in living cells by which energy is provided for vital processes and activities and new material is assimilated."

Therefore, the definition of metabolism is: *every single biochemical thing that happens in your body.* Every one of them!

Metabolism encompasses weight loss, but also muscle *building*, which would include weight gain. It also consists of the way in which your cells fight off disease, and how well they do that. That means your white blood cells and your immune cells work together to help you fight off and reverse disease and illness.

As I've mentioned before, your metabolism affects so much more than weight loss.

It affects:

- How well your heart functions
- How well your muscles create strength and activate freely
- How all your organs are working

The better all your cells are working — you have between fifty trillion and one hundred trillion of them — the better you're able to lose fat, build muscle, and stay healthy.

The Importance of Metabolism in Losing Fat, Building Muscle, and Fighting Disease

Let's talk about how important metabolism is to weight loss. You have a whole cascade of processes happening in your body that signal your fat cells to get smaller. That's what you want when you're trying to lose weight; you're trying to get your fat cells to shrink. It's your metabolism that's going to determine if, and how quickly, that is going to occur.

A lot of folks believe: *I can make my fat cells get smaller if I eat less.*

That's not always the case. What you're really trying to do is get your *adipose tissue* — those are your fat cells — to release their fatty acids and use those fatty acids as a form of energy.

Many people have been taught that fat cells get burned up; that's not really true. Fat cells go through a conversion process and release energy that you can use. The result is carbon dioxide and water. As I've mentioned before, many different cells in your body need to work in sequence for that to occur. This means your body must release these signals to your fat cells to release those fatty acids.

If these signals aren't released and received properly, you're not going to:

- Lose fat effectively
- Lose fat easily

If those fatty acids are released but aren't used, they'll end up right back where they started — in your fat cells.

If there is any kink in the chain, you won't be able to lose body fat.

It's so important to get your metabolism working solidly and to make sure every single process is working well. Remember: metabolism is the sum of all the biological processes in your body, so you need *all* the processes working at 100 percent and working 100 percent correctly for the changes in your body to occur the way you want them to.

Why Metabolism Is Important for Building Muscle

Again, keep in mind that metabolism is the sum of all the processes in your body — all of them — and this includes building muscle.

Have you ever had any trouble building muscle?

Do you know people who have had no problem building muscle?

If you look at the best bodybuilders in the world, they have the ability to build a lot of muscle *and* be extremely lean. That's no coincidence! Many people believe that genetics determine your ability to build muscle, and how quickly you can do it. Although it is true that there's a genetic influence, you can still create and build muscle regardless of your age or genetics.

You have the biological and physical ability to build muscle, based on your metabolism. The higher your metabolism, the faster you're going to build muscle. And the way you build muscle is with muscle-building exercise, of course. Muscle-building exercise helps you tear and break apart muscle, which is what signals your body to build more muscle. You need to have a healthy, functioning metabolism for that to work.

When your muscle cells get a little bit damaged by tearing and breaking apart, they release certain signals in your body, called *hormones*, to tell the muscle cells to grow and repair. Again, there are many different chemical processes involved that must happen in sequence for this to occur.

If there's a kink in that chain — if there's one set of cells that's not doing their job, or a muscle cell that's not receiving the correct signal — guess what's not going to happen?

The muscle cell is not going to grow. It's not going to get stronger. A healthy, highly functioning metabolism builds muscle quickly. The faster your metabolism, the faster you'll build muscle.

Fighting and Reversing Disease

Finally, let's talk about staying healthy, fighting disease, and reversing disease. Really, they're all the same thing.

The word *metabolism* comes from the Greek word *metabole*, which means *to change*. Metabolism is your body's ability to change. So when you're sick, your body has changed states. To fight sickness, it has to change to another state. Again, metabolism is the sum of all the biological processes in your body. When you're ill, your immune system launches an all-out assault against the foreign invaders that are creating sickness in your body and works to return it to health and equilibrium. The faster your metabolism does that, the faster it's able to fight off any sickness or illness that's in your body.

Have you ever noticed that sometimes you get a cold or a minor illness that lasts for days or possibly even weeks?

When you have a slow or low-functioning metabolism, not only does it take longer to lose weight and build muscle, but it also takes a lot longer for your body to return to good health.

When you have a fast or highly functioning metabolism, not only are you able to lose weight and build muscle quickly, but you also return to health very quickly.

When anyone in my family gets sick with the common cold — which happens a lot, especially with the children bringing home illnesses from being exposed to sick kids in their classrooms — sometimes we're only sick for as little as a few hours. Within eight to sixteen hours, we're back to 100 percent health again, which didn't happen when we had slower metabolisms. The same is true with fighting disease. The way your body reverses illness and disease is through a healthy metabolism. Your body is always trying to reverse disease. When you are providing your body with what it needs, and giving it what all your cells want, it will reverse disease. That is what it's programmed to do: to get back to optimal, functional health.

The only reason someone struggles with a disease is because they simply don't have the raw materials their cells need to be able to reverse that disease or to do what they need to get back to health. My wife, Dr. Brooke Goldner, was diagnosed with lupus, and we completely cured it. Her body was able to completely reverse a disease that's considered incurable, simply by fixing her metabolism.

One final note: The reason I am teaching you about metabolism is because this has unlocked the potential in my own ability—and that of countless students all over the world—to be able to lose weight and create strength, muscle, and tone faster and easier than was ever done in the past. It also saved my wife's life.

The Better Your Metabolism, the Faster Your Results

We all want to get the fastest, best results that we can in anything we do. Metabolism is the driver, the deciding factor, that determines how quickly and easily you get the results you want, whether it's fat loss, muscle gain, or improved health.

At this point, it's important to understand more deeply the impact of a fast metabolism and how it works. But I'm going to keep it simple at the same time. As I've mentioned, you have fifty trillion to one hundred trillion cells in your body. How well your body functions is determined by how well each of those cells is working. That's it. Everything that you are and can do physically is a result of the health or the unhealthiness of those cells. Disease is a result of how unhealthy some of those cells in your body are.

So how do you make these cells healthy?

How do you promote optimally functioning cells?

What's the difference between happy cells and unhealthy cells?

It's quite simple. The cells in your body are obedient little workers that make up who you are physically. They will do exactly what you tell them to, and they're very low maintenance. All they need to be able to do their job at 100 percent is simply the right raw materials. And each cell — *each* cell or each *type* of cell — has a different set of requirements of raw materials. For example, horses graze; lions eat meat; hummingbirds drink nectar, and so on. Food requirements for the species are not the same — they're different.

You've got the same process in your body. You've got different cells, and they need different nutrients. Your ability to get results is based on feeding every one of your cells the nutrients they need to be able to do their job. If you're trying to build a new addition to your house, your cells are like all the workers who are going to build that beautiful addition. The nutrients you give your body's cells are the same as the raw materials that you give your workers to build your home's new addition.

What most people do is focus on four things:

- Fat
- Carbohydrates
- Protein
- Water

That's the equivalent of saying, "I want you to build a beautiful, modern, state-of-the-art addition to our house, but all I'm going to give you is concrete, wood, and some spackle. That's it, nothing more."

A builder would never be able to construct an addition that way. They'd need a lot more materials! Roofing materials, nails, screws, wiring, pipes, paint, and so on. It's the same with your body. You can't just give it carbohydrates, protein, fat, and water. That's not even close to all the materials it needs. You need the full array of nutrients so you can:

- Completely feed all the cells in your body
- Build muscle
- Lose fat
- Be healthy

The better you feed your body the nutrients it needs, the better your metabolism will be and, therefore, the better your results in losing weight and building muscle.

All of this can be done through proper nutrition. It's all about your metabolism. Whenever you are frustrated with results, or any time you want a change to happen in your body, I want you always to focus on your metabolism.

SELF-TEST EVALUATION: DO YOU HAVE A SLOW METABOLISM? LET'S FIND OUT

The first step is to figure out how fast or slow your metabolism is.

A lot of folks believe that:

- People with a faster metabolism are always skinny.

- Younger people have a faster metabolism.
- Older people have a slower metabolism.

These statements are not always true. Plenty of people are able to stay thin. And although that can be a trait of a fast metabolism, it doesn't necessarily mean they have a fast metabolism.

Let's go over the symptoms of a slow metabolism. I want you to see firsthand if your metabolism needs improvement. In my experience, I've noticed that almost *everybody's* metabolism could use improvement and could be a lot faster than it is. So let's dive into the common traits of a slow metabolism. I want you to notice if you have *any* of these traits.

What Are the Common Symptoms of a Slow Metabolism?

1. A lot of exercise yields little to no results.

Have you ever tried to lose weight or build muscle?

You've probably exercised a lot to try to accomplish this. You might have done a lot of running, gone to the gym every single day, always worked up a great sweat, and you did this consistently for weeks. After a month or two, you looked at your results, and you had very little or nothing to show for it.

This reminds me of a time when I was on a P90X user forum. P90X is a top-selling home exercise program. It's solid from an exercise standpoint. One thing I noticed, though, is that the nutrition side of the program doesn't focus on metabolism. So, it works really well for people who already have a fast metabolism going in, but not so well for people who don't have a fast metabolism.

Here's what I mean: I went on the forum, and there was a gentleman who shared his thirty-day results with before-and-after pictures. When you looked at the pictures, you didn't see much difference at all.

The gentleman wrote, "Day thirty: no results."

Have you ever felt like that?

Have you ever gone through that experience?

Trust me, you're not alone. A lot of people try to lose weight, and they work really hard but don't have anything to show for their efforts. I know how frustrating that can be but don't worry. I know how to fix it.

If you have answered yes to this slow metabolism symptom, please mark it down. It's definitely a symptom of a slow metabolism.

2. A little bit of junk food equals big weight gain.

A long time ago, a woman named Kelly Clarkson won the first *American Idol* competition. If you look back at her pictures when she first went on *American Idol*, she looked a lot different than she does now. After she won, she had to do a lot of video and photo shoots, and she wanted to look good for America.

What did she do?

She got herself into shape. She worked with a personal trainer, went on a calorie- and carbohydrate-restricted diet—which most people do when they're trying to lose weight—and she lost a lot of inches and a lot of weight. She dropped quite a few sizes. She did her photo shoots, and she looked amazing. Then, after all the video and photo shoots were done, she went back to her old way of eating. She didn't change anything, she just went and ate the same diet as before—and suddenly, she blew up even bigger than the size she had been when she started. Imagine that!

Has this ever happened to you?

You lose weight and then go back to eating a little bit of junk food and—no matter how hard you exercise or work out—suddenly, almost all the weight comes back. It's almost as if you didn't make any progress at all, just because of one small bout of eating junk food.

If that describes you, it's another symptom of a slow metabolism, so please mark it down.

3. No matter what you do, your problem areas never go away.

I'm sure you have some problem areas on your body that you wish would just improve or go away. If you don't, that's wonderful. But if you do, that's okay; know that you're not alone. There are some common problem areas a lot of women share. I know this because I used to own and operate one of the largest indoor fitness boot camps in Orange County, California. More than 90 percent of our members were women, and they would complain about the same thing.

Maybe you have the same problem areas:

- The roll of fat around your belly
- Flat buttocks
- Flabby triceps/back of the upper arms

For both men and women, the area around the waist can be a problem—no matter how many sit-ups you do, no matter how much you run and how often you work out.

Do you ever work out consistently and go on a diet for weeks and weeks, and you're able to lose some weight, but still, when you look down, you can grab a roll of fat around your belly?

It never seems to get toned and defined. It stays soft, despite your efforts. That might be a medical condition I made up, known as *pooch-itis*. Don't worry — that's a symptom of a slow metabolism, and we can fix that.

Men like to work the upper body, and are able to get muscular pretty easily, or at least a lot quicker than women do, because of their higher levels of anabolic hormones. But despite all the sit-ups and crunches they do, they still have a beer belly. If that's you, chances are you have a slow metabolism as well, and I'll tell you exactly how to fix it.

Another problem area I hear about a lot is flat buttocks.

Have you noticed that the Brazilian butt-lift seems to be a big fitness fad right now?

A lot of women are trying to get that nice, toned, rounded butt, so they do leg exercises, donkey-kick exercises, squats, and lunges, and they'll use the stairs for weeks and weeks. But after a few months, they look at their results, and their backsides are still flat.

Has that ever happened to you?

You can't seem to build more roundness and firmness in your tush?

That probably just means that you have a slow metabolism, and I know exactly how to fix that.

How about the backs of your arms?

A client came to me, lifted her arms and pointed to her triceps. She asked, "How do I get rid of these batwings?"

She told me that she did all the exercises for triceps almost every time she went to the gym, but after several weeks there was no improvement. She lifted her arms up, and her upper arms sagged.

She said, "They flap in the wind. How do you fix that?"

I said, "Well, you have to raise your metabolism. We can trim that up."

If you're suffering from a problem area like that, chances are you have a slow metabolism, too.

4. **Whenever you get sick, the sickness lasts for a** *long* **time.**

Have you ever had a common cold or gotten sick?

How long did it take you to fully, 100 percent recover?

Was it just a few hours?

A few days?

A few weeks?

If it's taken you more than a few days to fully recover from the common cold, then you have a symptom of a slow metabolism. Here's why: I didn't realize how quickly the human body is able to get over sickness and illness until I raised my metabolism myself, and I was able to compare my recovery to what it had been before.

I was able to look at my wife's results, too, and compare her speed of recovery versus what it used to be before she had a fast metabolism. Our children go to school, which is often a cesspool of disease and sickness, especially during the winter. My kids would catch colds from the other children, and then they would pass them onto us. It used to take me at least four or five days to get over a cold, maybe even a couple weeks, and now it only takes me just one or two days, tops, before I'm back to complete, 100 percent health.

It's the same with my wife. As I've mentioned before, she had an autoimmune disease that meant that whenever she had a cold, it would last sometimes weeks. With a higher metabolism, she's able to get back to complete health within a day or two, maximum. Whenever our children are sick, they're healthy again within a day or two.

If you notice you are slow to recover from illness, there's a chance you have a slow metabolism, so please mark it down.

The Self-Test Evaluation

Out of the four symptoms of a slow metabolism, if you've said yes to *any* of those symptoms, you possibly have a slower metabolism than you could. This is great news, because it means there are things you can do to raise your metabolism. I want you to get excited about this, because it means that you're going to be able to get faster results.

What Happens When You Have a Slow Metabolism?

Nicole came to me as a client many years ago to help get her pre-pregnancy body back. As a mother of four children, she felt *frumpy* — her own word — unsexy, and old. Plus, the weight she had gained during the pregnancies hadn't all gone away. She was frustrated with being unable to fit into her favorite skinny jeans that she wore before she had her first child. She wanted to lose weight, shrink her waist, and feel sexy, young, and beautiful again.

She said, "My overall goal is to lose weight. I would like to lose four inches from my waist. Although I need to lose weight all over, the weight around my middle is what I dislike the most. I have four children, and I have not had a flat stomach since my first pregnancy ten years ago."

Luckily, I told her, she came to the right place, because my Boot Camp was known for achieving some of the fastest weight-loss results out there. But it only really, truly works—just like any other exercise program does, even the P90X—if you combine it with a diet that raises your metabolism. She said she was fine with her diet; she was eating 1,200 calories or less a day, and said she didn't need any help with that.

I said, "Okay, I can't guarantee the results, but let's see what we can do."

Nicole came in religiously, five days a week, and worked out really hard. After three months, she reported back to me.

"I have been losing weight slowly but surely since starting the Boot Camp fitness program. I have lost ten pounds in three months," she said.

She went on to tell me that, despite losing ten pounds, she hadn't lost any inches from her waist, nor did she drop any pants or dress sizes. First I congratulated her, and then calculated her monthly rate of results.

What do you think her monthly rate of results were, in terms of weight?

I'll make it easy for you. It was 3.3 pounds per month.

Do you think those are good results?

Are those results comparable to what you're getting right now when trying to lose weight, or are they different?

In my world, those results are way too slow.

I said to Nicole, "I have a suspicion that you have a slow metabolism, and that's why you have not been able to get your pre-pregnancy body back, despite all the work you're doing. Let's see what we can do. Let's take a closer look at what's going on with your diet, and let's confirm if you have a slow metabolism or not."

LET'S START RAISING YOUR METABOLISM TO-DAY

In the previous section, you learned what a slow metabolism is and what happens when you have a slow metabolism. If you have any of the four symptoms of a slow metabolism, it means that your metabolism is slower than what you could potentially have.

Let's start raising your metabolism today, so that you can have:

- Faster weight-loss results
- Faster fat-loss results
- Faster muscle-building results
- Faster recovery from illness

- Stronger immune system, so it's hard to get sick in the first place

You'll be amazed at how quickly you'll be able to create the results you want in your body and in your health once you raise your metabolism! Let's get started doing that in this section.

Fast-Metabolism Meals

Because your metabolism is 100 percent dependent on the health of the trillions of cells in your body, what it boils down to is making sure you feed those trillions of cells exactly what they need, so they can do their jobs. Let's go over a proven template for how to drastically raise your metabolism by feeding all the cells in your body.

The main trait of a fast-metabolism nutrition plan is that you *do not* focus on what to take away from your body. That's what all the other diets do; they focus on what to take away. Your metabolism is reduced when you take food away. You want to raise your metabolism, so what we're going to focus on is putting in what your body is missing. I want you to sit back and be amazed at the results. Here are the components of a fast-metabolism diet.

1. A fast-metabolism diet is extremely high in nutrient-dense foods.

Nutrient-dense foods are extremely high in vitamins, minerals, and *phytonutrients*, or plant nutrients that are especially good at maintaining our health and vitality.

What are the most abundant nutrient-dense foods?

Most important, produce; and more specifically, vegetables. Vegetables, by far, have the highest vitamin, mineral, phytonutrient, and nutrient content of all the foods, and the best part about it is they can all be found in your grocery store. Highly nutrient-dense, whole foods are one of the biggest keys to a fast metabolism, and you should eat them in large amounts.

Seventy-five percent or more of your diet should come from high-nutrient, whole foods. If you're consuming less than that, it could be a reason your metabolism isn't as fast as you want it to be.

2. A fast-metabolism diet has a high amount of omega-3s.

Omega-3s are one of the most important nutrients in your body. Omega-3s are a type of fat that most of us don't get enough of.

They are responsible for many functions in your body:

- They are the raw materials that make up the walls of every cell in your body.

- They are responsible for the myelin sheath around all the nerves in your brain and throughout your body.

- They help your brain function well.

- They help the efficient and productive creation of hormones in the body.

- They allow your fat and muscle cells to receive the signals to shrink and grow effectively.

- Omega-3s are the components that help make your cells fluid and flexible, and able to perform their functions at 100 percent effectiveness.

If you're getting anything less than a handful of whole chia seeds or flaxseeds, you are probably slowing down your metabolism. Let's increase your intake of omega-3s so you can raise your metabolism.

3. **The final, most important component of raising your metabolism is water.**

You need to have a lot of water. There are a lot of books and information available that help you try to estimate your ideal water intake. I've seen many of them, and I am going to present to you, simply, what has worked 100 percent of the time from my experience. Anything less than ninety-six ounces of pure water a day seems to slow down metabolism and slow down results. Make sure you're getting at least ninety-six ounces of water *every single day*, because every single biological process in the body happens via the medium of water.

If you don't have enough water in your body, you're slowing down your metabolism. Some of the chemical processes in your body can't even happen if you don't have enough water. That includes being able to properly — *properly* — lose fat and build muscle. Without enough water, everything in your body slows down. So let's speed them up and make sure you're getting at least ninety-six ounces of water every day.

Sample Fast-Metabolism Meal

- Steamed kale and mushrooms
- A few sprays of Bragg Liquid Aminos
- Nutritional yeast sprinkled on top
- Fresh avocado
- Fresh-cut tomato

Fast-Metabolism Smoothies

Now that we've discussed how to increase your metabolism through your diet, how would you like a way to get all those wonderful, fast-metabolism foods without having to worry about making all your meals and preparing something that's delicious and something gourmet, which requires time and effort?

How would you like to be able to get all these nutrients in less than five minutes?

Your blender is going to be one of your best friends.

When I tell clients about the fast-metabolism meals, they say, "I don't have the time to make all these meals! I don't like to cook. I'm not good in the kitchen."

I say, "Great, then you are going to *love* fast-metabolism smoothies!"

If you don't have the time or don't feel like investing the time making these meals, that is fine. You can just put all those ingredients into a high-powered blender, like a Vitamix or Blendtec, turn it on, and two minutes later, you have a wonderfully amazing, delicious, and highly nutritious fast-metabolism smoothie, which you can drink in just a few seconds.

A lot of folks wonder, "Is that enough to eat?"

I say usually you can eat *more* and get more in your body using the smoothies than you can by chewing. It's the same ingredients, but it's just been pre-chewed a little bit by the blender. I love smoothies, because smoothies allow me to make my meals quickly, efficiently, conveniently, and bring them with me everywhere I go.

Let me share a few of my favorite fast-metabolism smoothies that you can make yourself to make raising your metabolism even easier.

Below is a step-by-step template to make it easier for you to create your own custom fast-metabolism smoothies.

The amounts given are in percentages, relative to the total amount of food ingredients in the blender container, not including ice, water, and nut milk.

Step 1: add 75 percent or more nutrient-dense, raw vegetables.

Awesome Fast-Metabolism Vegetables:

Asparagus	Lettuce
Bok Choy	Kale
Beets	Onion
Beet greens	Parsley
Broccoli	Peppers
Brussels sprouts	Radish
Cabbage	Spinach
Carrots	Squash

Cauliflower	Sweet potato
Celery	Swiss chard
Collard greens	Turnip
Cucumber	Zucchini

Step 2: add 25 percent or less of fruits and fats.

Flavorful Fruits:

Apples	Oranges
Bananas	Pears
Berries	Tomatoes
Grapes	

Fat-Burning Fats

Chia seeds

Flaxseeds

Step 3: add as much liquid as you like from these sources.

Refreshing Fillers:

Almond milk

Hemp milk

Rice milk

Water

Step 4 (optional): add any superfoods you like.

Super Foods

> Spirulina
> Chlorella
> Maca

Basically, you're going to combine the fast-metabolism vegetables, favorite fast-metabolism fruits, favorite fast-metabolism omega-3s, and then the different nut milks and waters. This is also a good opportunity to add any supplements, vitamins, extra vitamins, or superfoods as well. They go well in your smoothie and if you don't like the taste, that's perfect because the smoothie hides the taste.

Super Spinach Smoothie

> Lots of spinach
> 1 ripe banana
> 1 avocado
> Flaxseed oil
> Almond milk
> Water
> Ice cubes

Fill 60 to 75 percent of your blender with spinach and pack it down tight. Add a banana, an avocado, and a squirt of flaxseed oil (1–2 tbsp.). Then pour in about 1 cup of almond milk and fill the blender to about ¾ full with water. Top off with ice cubes and turn the blender on. Let it blend on high for about 2 minutes or until you get a nice consistency.

Fat-Killer Kale Smoothie

> Lots of kale
> 1 tart green apple
> 1 avocado
> Flaxseed oil
> Almond milk
> Water
> Ice cubes

Fill 60 to 75 percent of your blender with kale and pack it down tight. If the kale stems are spicy and bitter, remove them first. Add a green apple, an avocado, and a squirt of flaxseed oil (1-2 tbsp.). Then pour in about 1 cup of almond milk and fill the blender to about ¾ full with water. Top off with ice cubes and turn the blender on. Let it blend on high for about 2 minutes or until you get a nice consistency.

Beet Me Health Smoothie

> Black kale
> Celery
> Carrots

Raw beets
1 pear
Chia seeds
Chlorella
Spirulina
Water
Ice cubes

Fill 60 to 75 percent of your blender with an equal combination of black kale, celery, carrots, and raw beets. Add a pear and a small handful of chia seeds. Add a dash of chlorella and spirulina. Then fill about ¾ full with water and top it off with ice cubes. Turn the blender on and let it blend on high for about 2 minutes or until you get a nice consistency.

Fall for the Greens Smoothie

Kale
Parsley
Carrots
1 red apple
Flaxseed oil
Spirulina
Ice cubes
Water

Fill 60 to 75 percent of your blender with an equal combination of kale, parsley, and carrots. Add a red apple and a squirt of flaxseed oil (1-2 tbsp.). Add a dash of spirulina. Then fill about ¾ full with water and top it off with ice cubes. Turn the blender on and let it blend on high for about 2 minutes or until you get a nice consistency.

Super Green Smoothie

> Zucchini
> Persian cucumbers
> Spinach
> Mint leaves
> 1 avocado
> Flaxseed oil
> Ice cubes
> Water

Fill 60 to 75 percent of your blender with an equal combination of zucchini, Persian cucumbers, spinach, and mint leaves. Add an avocado and a squirt of flaxseed oil (1–2 tbsp.). Then fill about ¾ full with water and top it off with ice cubes. Turn the blender on and let it blend on high for about 2 minutes or until you get a nice consistency.

Thomas's Favorite Smoothie

> Lots of spinach
> Sweet grapes

3 ripe bananas
1 avocado
Ice cubes
Water

Fill 60 percent of your blender with spinach and pack it in tight. Add the bananas and avocado. Fill about 15 percent of the blender with the sweetest grapes you can buy. Pour in water until it reaches about ¾ full and top it off with ice cubes. Turn the blender on and let it blend on high for about 2 minutes or until you get a nice consistency.

Try these different smoothies and find the ones you like the most. The goal is to have at least two that you absolutely love. In case you don't, play around with the ingredients until you find a combination that creates a smoothie you find absolutely irresistible.

This is important, because the more delicious the smoothies are, the more likely you will be motivated to make them.

Case Studies

Remember my client Nicole, whom I mentioned in the previous section?

Her goal was to lose four inches from her waist and get her pre-pregnancy body back after having four children. She had just spent three months doing my Boot Camp, and eating a 1,200-calorie or less diet. She was only able to lose a total of ten pounds, with no inches from her waist gone, and no decrease in pants or dress sizes at all.

I told her, "Well, Nicole, you only lost an average of 3.3 pounds per month, which is very slow compared to what our average student loses, especially at your age and without our fast-metabolism nutrition. What do you think about us taking a look at what you're eating and seeing if it's your metabolism that's keeping you from getting the results you want?"

She agreed and shared with us her average diet for a day. Here's what it included:

Breakfast (7:30)

> Nonfat latte
> Kashi Go Lean cereal with milk or yogurt
> Poached egg on English muffin

Lunch (noon)

> Roasted turkey, cheese, and avocado sandwich
> Diet Coke

Dinner (7:00)

> Roasted chicken
> Vegetables
> 32 oz. water

At first glance, it looked like a pretty sensible diet, one that the average person would use. It was low calorie (in fact, the diet she submitted to me was less than 1,100 calories a day), it was lower on the carbohydrate side, and it's what most people generally do.

Now, let's break it down.

Is her diet high or low in fast-metabolism nutrients and nutrient-dense whole foods?

Is her diet high or low in omega-3s?

In other words, is she getting at least a handful of omega-3s from our favorite sources?

And is her diet high or low in water?

Is she getting at least ninety-six ounces of water a day?

The answers, of course, are low to no whole foods and high nutrient-dense foods; almost no omega-3s; and her water intake—only thirty-two ounces—is way below what she really needs.

This confirmed that Nicole was eating a slow-metabolism diet, so her metabolism was definitely slower than it could be.

I told Nicole, "We can fix this. We're going to put you on a fast-metabolism diet."

And here's what's wonderful: whenever I coach my high-end clients, we set up a scoreboard, because guidelines don't seem to work as effectively as a scoreboard does. People seem to work well when they get points and they understand the rules of the game.

Nicole needed to earn five points a day. She could get points by:

- Working out at the Boot Camp, which was already part of her routine (1 point)

- Consuming three fast-metabolism smoothies a day—she was a mother of four, and she was really busy, so smoothies were going to be her best friend (1 point)

- Consuming two fast-metabolism meals in addition to the smoothies; Nicole preferred big salads, which was fine (1 point)

- Drinking at least ninety-six ounces of water a day (1 point)

- Consuming omega-3s—at least a handful of flaxseeds or chia seeds (1 point)

Her goal every day was to score five points. If she was still hungry after earning those five points, she could continue eating all her previous foods as desired. However, the five points had to come first. Notice that we didn't take anything away. We just added nutrient-dense food and water.

Nicole did this for sixty straight days. *Sixty straight days.*

Let's compare what her results were after sixty days on her previous diet with exercise, and sixty days with the same exercise, but using the fast-metabolism diet. Her rate of results previously was 3.3 pounds per month. On average, in those sixty days she lost 6.6 pounds, zero inches off her waist, and zero change in her pants size.

After sixty days of using the fast-metabolism diet, and keeping everything else exactly the same, she lost 17.9 pounds. Her waist shrunk by 4.5 inches.

Remember she only wanted to lose four inches from her waist?

We exceeded her goals in just sixty days! Her pants size dropped two sizes within the same sixty days.

She wrote to me, "I'm fitting into clothes I haven't been able to wear for ages! I look better than I did when I left [another country]! Everything looks better!"

I have heard countless stories just like this one from clients who replaced their outdated, ineffective, and frustrating low-calorie, low-carbohydrate diets with this easy, healthy, and no-sacrifice fast-metabolism diets. They got the best results they'd seen in years, and for many, in their entire lives.

Nicole was able to wear all the clothes she loved so much, which had been collecting dust in her closet for more than ten years. This was the first time since her first pregnancy—for the first time in a decade—she was finally able to wear them again. What she also mentioned was how fun it was to be able to walk into a clothing store, pick out any outfit she wanted, and be excited by how good it looked on her. Before, she was depressed right before she had to go into a dressing room, every single time. Now, she doesn't have to worry about that anymore.

Action Plan

Let's make this happen for you. Let's start raising your metabolism right now. First things first: let's get your fast-metabolism meals and fast-metabolism smoothies ready to go, so you can easily raise your metabolism.

1. Build your ultimate salad.

I don't mean the bland, tasteless, pre-dinner salad you get at restaurants. We're not going to do that. I love using a base of romaine lettuce, spinach, and often kale for my salads. I put in lots of chopped broccoli, cucumber, palm hearts, artichokes, organic baby corn, cherry tomatoes, avocado, tangerine, apple chunks, and walnuts.

Then I top it all off with a fruit-based, homemade dressing that you can make in your blender. You can make up any combination that you want. Use any of the ingredients from the previous sections to experiment a little bit, and find what you love most. You can throw in a handful of raspberries, mix in a splash of almond milk to give it a creamy texture and consistency, and then pour it over your salad. I like the citrusy kinds of salad dressing.

My wife, Dr. Brooke Goldner, has an easy-to-make raw almond Caesar dressing recipe to die for.

The Doctor's Raw Almond Caesar Salad Dressing

Ingredients:

> 1 cup raw almonds
> 3 tbsp. lemon juice
> 2 tbsp. Bragg Liquid Aminos
> 2 tbsp. Dijon
> 3 cloves garlic
> 1/3 cup fortified nutritional yeast
> 1 ½ cup (approx.) filtered water

To prepare:

> Start with a cup of water and blend in power blender with all the other ingredients. Keep adding water until you like the consistency. Use what you want and store leftovers in the fridge. You'll need to add more water the next day as it thickens overnight.

2. Stock up on organic fruits and vegetables.

Did you ever have the impulse to eat something that you shouldn't?

If you have these wonderful fruits and vegetables ready to go, right in your refrigerator or pantry, there's a good chance that when you're going around hunting for food, you'll choose one of these rather than a less healthy choice.

Remember this: Convenience trumps all, so the more convenient a food is to eat, right then and there, the more likely you'll be to gravitate toward that food. Let's make your healthy, faster metabolism foods the most convenient options. Have some fruits and chopped-up organic vegetables ready to go in your fridge or out in the open at all times.

3. Get some omega-3s.

Omega-3s are amazing when it comes to raising metabolism. Our favorite sources of omega-3s are whole flaxseeds and chia seeds. We do not recommend ground flaxseeds or chia seeds. Once they are ground, the omega-3s begin to oxidize, making them useless. Flaxseeds and chia seeds are very cheap and can be found online and at any grocery store.

4. To make it super easy, fill a whole gallon jug of water.

Although you only need ninety-six ounces, go ahead and fill the entire gallon. A trick that many professional bodybuilders use is to fill up an entire gallon container with water, and then they just make it a goal to finish it by the end of the day.

There's a saying: "Out of sight, out of mind."

When you fill up a gallon jug and you drag it around with you, it's always in sight, which means you always keep water on your mind.

Be warned: If you're not used to drinking a gallon of water a day, you will pee a lot more frequently in the beginning. But believe me, your body's going to get used to it. You're going to be more hydrated, have better energy, and raise your metabolism as a result. It is worth it, and you will get used to it. Plus, there's nothing wrong with burning a few extra calories and getting a little bit more movement in your day by getting up and going to the bathroom and back.

In the next chapter, we'll discuss more ways to raise your metabolism with the help of an amazing tool that's going to make your fast-metabolism diet the easiest and most results-getting body transformation strategy ever!

CHAPTER TWO

The Metabolic Miracle—
Healing From Disease

**THE TOP *HEALTHY* FOODS THAT ARE HURTING
YOUR HEALTH**

It's important that you become aware of what foods
you're eating right now that are actually slowing down
your metabolism and hurting your health. One thing
you must understand is that all the food you eat impacts
your health. You also must understand that metabolism
equals health. The better your metabolism, the better
your health. But also, the worse your metabolism, the
worse your health. Let's go over some of the most
common so-called *healthy* foods that actually have a
negative effect on your health and metabolism.

Dairy

I remember when I was growing up, hearing those ads
on TV saying, "Milk: It does a body good. Milk has lots
of calcium, and calcium is good for strong bones."

I had always associated milk with giving me a lot of strength, making my bones healthy, and helping me build a lot of muscle, because they also say that milk is high in protein. Later in life, I also had learned that milk is low-glycemic, which means that milk supposedly is released as sugar in your bloodstream more slowly than other foods. Therefore, the claim is that milk and all other dairy products, including yogurt and cheese, help you lose weight. These foods have always been recommended, because they're supposedly healthy.

We now know—through proven science, research, and millions of human case studies—that milk is actually the opposite of all those things. And it's highly toxic—milk doesn't do a body good, because *milk causes inflammation*. Studies done by Colin Campbell, professor of nutrition at Cornell University, show that milk is a cancer switch: when you drink milk or eat dairy products, you're increasing the rate at which cancer can grow in your body, and you're also rapidly raising your chances of getting cancer. (nutritionstudies.org)

Although milk is low-glycemic, which means that the sugar from milk is released more slowly in your body than other foods, it is highly *insulinemic*, which means that it raises your insulin level higher than just about any other food. Consuming dairy products like milk, yogurt, and cheese raises insulin, which is the hormone that directly causes you to store fat. Dairy raises insulin levels higher than even white bread, which we all know is not good for losing weight.

And though we've been told that we need the calcium in milk to create strong bones, the exact opposite is true. The calcium in milk is not the kind of calcium that's easily absorbed by the human body. Milk and all dairy products are highly acidic, which means that they lower the pH in your body, which is toxic for your body. Your body responds by releasing calcium from your bones to raise the pH so that you're healthy again.

In other words, consuming milk and dairy products weakens your bones and promotes osteoporosis. So, if you're drinking milk, or eating yogurt or cheese, thinking that you're doing something good for your body, please know that you're not. Dairy is one of the first things I recommend you take out of your diet as quickly as possible so that you can increase your metabolism and also improve your health.

Finally, the protein from milk comes from casein. Many bodybuilders like to talk about casein as a great, slow-releasing protein that's good for the body. Numerous studies have shown that casein itself is a cancer switch. Studies have shown, not just in laboratory animals but also in humans, that consuming casein causes inflammation, which is a cause of cancer. One more thing, from my wife, Dr. Brooke Goldner: casein is a cancer promoter on a DNA level. It attaches at the promoter region and tells the cells to create cancer cells by activating the cancer genes. Dairy literally and physically turns on cancer genes.

Meat

The second most common food promoted as healthy is meat.

Many folks, when they're trying to eat clean or get healthy, say, "I'm going to avoid the red meat, and instead I'm just going to eat the white meat."

So they eat lots of seafood, fish, and chicken. Based on research and human experience, the reality is that all meat causes illness. Consuming meat causes *inflammation* in the body. Inflammation is the body's response to any sort of injury or illness. Our bodies wouldn't get inflamed if we weren't eating something toxic, and meat is highly toxic. Whether it's chicken, fish, or beef, all meat can cause cancer. All of it can increase insulin levels and cause diabetes. And it can cause weight gain because of the effect on insulin levels. All meat can cause inflammation, which also leads to high cholesterol and heart disease.

Many people eat meat as a source of protein. I am going to show you, in the next few chapters, how you can get all the protein you could ever want from nonmeat sources that will not increase inflammation, and in fact, will decrease inflammation instead, improving your health and raising your metabolism at the same time.

If you consume meat in any form, you are risking your health. Also, you are not absorbing all of the protein you could be absorbing, because when you raise your levels of inflammation, you also lower your ability to absorb the amino acids from the protein that you're eating. Studies have shown that more than half the protein you consume from animal products does not get absorbed. In the next few chapters, I'll show you how you can get your protein from different sources and absorb *all* of it, without the negative health effects.

Processed Foods

The last most common food that many people eat, especially when they are trying to get healthy, are processed foods, especially the so-called *healthy* foods.

Have you ever seen ads for Special K or Go Lean cereals, in which they're promoted as healthy options for losing weight and improving health?

Well, those turn out to be some of the worst foods you could eat.

Why is that?

Because they're highly processed.

What does that mean?

Processed foods are:

- Refined (milled down) from their naturally grown state
- Bleached
- Stripped of certain nutrients
- Combined with chemicals

What is left is simply edible matter that usually raises your insulin, increasing your chance of diabetes, and can raise your cholesterol, as well as a whole host of other things.

Almost all processed foods — just like meat and dairy:

- Raise inflammation, which increases your risk of cancer and heart disease, among many other illnesses
- Increase your susceptibility for illness
- Lower your metabolism
- Make it harder to lose weight

The truth is, when you're eating Go Lean cereal with milk, you have created a cocktail for weight gain. And that's exactly what you *don't* want to do if your goal is to get leaner, fitter, and healthier as quickly as possible.

Processed foods include cereals, most breads, and most carbohydrate-based products. If it comes in a box, I guarantee it's a processed food. If it's not produce, and it doesn't look the same as when it came out of the ground or was plucked from a tree, it's a processed food. It had to go through some sort of processing to become what it is. Anything that has a shelf life of more than four to five days is probably processed.

Think about it: how long can raw fruits and vegetables live after they've been harvested?

I guarantee it's not as long as processed food. Many boxed, processed foods—like pastas, breads, and cereals—can live on a shelf for an unlimited amount of time. There's nothing living in those processed foods. It is all dead, edible matter, and that's it.

What About Nuts and Seeds?

Although nuts and seeds have long shelf lives and aren't processed, they still don't contain near the nutrient density of produce. Nuts and seeds need to germinate and begin to form a plant in order to unlock their nutrients. The primary nutrient we seek from seeds like flaxseeds and chia seeds are the anti-inflammatory omega-3s. Nearly all nuts and seeds are a rich source of fatty acids, most of them pro-inflammatory omega-6 fatty acids. That is why we prefer flaxseeds and chia seeds to all other nuts and seeds.

CURING AN INCURABLE DISEASE – BROOKE'S STORY

I never expected to be writing a book like this. After I met the love of my life, I found out she had an incurable disease. The sadness I experienced, knowing I was not going to be able to grow old or have children with my soul mate, was absolutely devastating. When we accidentally stumbled upon the cure, I knew it was my life's mission to get this information to as many people as possible. We discovered that not only was the cure for her disease achievable, but it also was the key to improved health and fitness. You can use this information to not only give yourself the body of your dreams, but also share and help the people in your life who you care about, as well.

Inflammation: The Root Cause of Most Disease

Inflammation is a term describing the immune system's response to illness and disease. Inflammation is on the rise because of the foods most of us eat. When we get sick, inflammation in our body tries to fight the sickness. Whenever we are injured or hurt, we see a bruise or swelling, which is inflammation. But when we consume foods that are toxic to our bodies, the inflammation starts from within our blood vessels, lungs, brain, and organs. Cancer, heart disease, and diabetes are all inflammatory diseases.

As I've mentioned before, my wife had lupus—an inflammatory disease, at a very young age. When I met my wife, we were both twenty-eight. She told me that because of the lupus she wasn't going to live very long, maybe to her mid-forties.

She said, "By my mid- or late thirties, you're going to have to start taking care of me, because even right now, I'm taking medicine and shots just to protect my brain from blood clots. I'm not going to be able to have children. It's certain death. If I try to have a child, I'm going to die, and it's going to kill the baby as well."

All I wanted was to be with Brooke, my soul mate, and I decided to marry her anyway, knowing she had all these medical issues. But I hoped and prayed that there was some way we could spend a few more extra years together. We focused on living a healthy lifestyle and doing what we could to be as fit as we could, to live in the time left the best way possible.

Lupus is a disease in which the body turns against itself, because the inflammation is so high and so chronic. With this inflammation, your cells can't function normally. They kind of go haywire and don't do their job the way they're supposed to. The body's cells turn on themselves, and they start attacking your own body, thinking parts of your own body—your organs—are the illness or are foreign invaders. This is how lupus eventually kills you. It's also considered an incurable disease; there's no medicine, or anything known by Western medicine, to cure lupus.

Living with Lupus

Every morning, I'd wake up and see Brooke in the bathroom, giving herself a shot. Every time I saw that, it broke my heart because I knew that I had one less day with her, and I knew that I didn't have very many. She needed those shots, because they were protecting her from having a stroke. With lupus, high inflammation promotes blood clots, which can circulate through your body and eventually flow up to your brain. If it gets stuck in one of the blood vessels or capillaries in your brain, you have a stroke.

I remember Brooke telling me a story about when she was going through medical school, and she had what was called a mini-stroke, or *transient ischemic attack* (TIA), which is a temporary stroke. There was a blood clot moving through her brain; it stopped temporarily, but thank goodness it kept going. A mini-stroke could have resulted in permanent brain damage, and possibly affected her for the rest of her life. Luckily it didn't, but that's how devastating lupus can be.

After a while, lupus patients start experiencing other symptoms and conditions, such as arthritis, and they can't move their joints and limbs very well, because they're in constant pain. They can't be out in the sun very much, because that causes the lupus to flare, putting them at risk of becoming very sick and putting their lives at risk. We had to make sure we stayed out of the sun. We also had to make sure we didn't think about having babies, because that's an automatic death wish right there, and a whole host of other things. Just day-to-day life was so difficult and required so much work. The scariest part was knowing that all of it would come to an end very soon. That's what it felt like to live with lupus.

All I wanted, every day, was just to live an extra day with the love of my life. I would do and give anything to have more time with her.

How We Accidentally Cured It

It took only three weeks for us to fall madly in love with each other.

I said, "Let's get married!"

She looked at me and said, "Are you sure you want to marry me?"

I said, "Of course!"

I was kind of shocked — why was she asking me that?

She told me about the lupus, and what it meant. I was shocked and stunned to suddenly learn that the love of my life had a terminal disease that would take her life in the next ten to fifteen years.

"Why?" I cried to myself.

At that moment, I had to make a decision.

Do I say, *yes*, and voluntarily face what could be the greatest loss of my life?

Or do I say, *no* and miss the greatest love I've ever known?

I said, "I'd rather live a short life with you than a lifetime with anyone else. If it's going to be a short life, it's going to be the best life you ever had!"

Brooke said, "Okay, well, I want to look hot for my wedding!"

I said, "Well, you married the right guy."

At the time, Brooke was a size 10, and she wanted to get down to a size 6 or size 4.

I said, "Okay, I've got the perfect plan for you."

I put her on a ninety-day program, which consisted of incredibly high amounts of living, raw vegetables, and produce. Brooke was a vegetarian at the time, so she preferred to get her protein mostly from plant sources. I put her on a rigorous fitness regimen, which was an hour or two of exercise, six days a week.

After ninety days, she had the body of her dreams! She dropped from a size 10 to a size 4, and she was stronger, leaner, and more toned than she'd ever been. She had toned her stomach, which was something she had always wanted. We decided to have our wedding in Hawaii. She looked better than she had ever looked, and we got to take the most beautiful pictures of her in her bathing suit and in her bridal gown. We came back and started our life together, even though we knew it was going to be a short one.

We were changing doctors, so Brooke needed to get a checkup. The doctor wanted to get a full scope of blood work to see how the lupus was progressing. When we got the test results back, there was no lupus in her body! When that happens, it usually means that the lab got blood tests mixed up with someone else's.

The doctor said, "This is impossible. It must have been a mix-up, so we need to do a retest."

She was retested, and a month later we got the results. Not only was the lupus completely gone from her body, but also her health was perfect. Her overall health was at the same level as an elite athlete. At that point, we looked at each other, and we didn't think we had stumbled upon a cure—we just thought we had gotten lucky!

We continued living the same way we had previously, because Brooke enjoyed the way she looked and felt, eating the diet I advised her to eat. And she loved being fit, so she continued working out. Little did we know that those were the factors that had cured the lupus.

A year after we were married, she was off all lupus medications, and her blood work still showed absolutely no sign of lupus. Then we started spending some time in the sun, in the middle of the day. Again, no lupus was showing up, even though we were playing in the sun day after day.

A year later, Brooke said something to me that I thought was absolutely crazy.

She said, "I want a baby."

We both knew full well that getting pregnant was something that killed lupus patients.

I said, "Are you crazy?"

She said, "No, I'm serious. I want a baby and I think I can do it!"

Then her mother jumped in and said, "I'll have the baby."

I said, "No! That would be really wrong."

Then I found out that you can use in vitro fertilization — no physical relations required.

But either way, we said, "Okay, you know what? Let's give it a shot."

Brooke promised me if anything came up in any blood tests or checkups that put her or the baby in danger, she would do whatever she needed to be safe.

We finally got pregnant. Tensions were high among the family. Brooke was going in for her checkups with a high-risk obstetrician, and they did rigorous testing on her. As the baby grew and the pregnancy progressed, there was no sign at all of lupus, and her health was stellar.

She gave birth to our first son, Solomon, and it was a flawless birth. Brooke was back on her feet the same day, and our baby was completely healthy. Brooke's health was never affected; the lupus never came back despite the doctors' predictions that the lupus would return during the pregnancy.

None of that happened, and we finally said to ourselves, "We are onto something here. We need to figure out what we did, because we cured this disease."

Brooke and I realized that the only thing different in her life was simply going on my fitness and nutrition program, the ninety-day dream body program. We began to reverse-engineer my diet and fitness program to understand what it was about those two things that had a positive effect on her health and cured the lupus. After a year and a half of tearing through volumes of biochemistry books and research abstracts, we figured it out.

Since then, we launched a best-selling book, *Goodbye Lupus*, and an online medical practice. We have been helping countless patients completely reverse their lupus and numerous autoimmune diseases with nothing more than the fast metabolism diet.

There's a good chance you picked up this book because you want to get healthier, lose weight, or build muscle and strength. But what this is really about is honoring yourself and your body, and following your heart. It's impossible to know ahead of time the miracles that are going to happen when you pursue your own health. Whether it's for yourself or someone else, the amazing miracles that happen in every aspect of your life occur when you truly start to honor your health, your body, and yourself.

Treating your body with respect is one of the greatest ways to honor yourself as a person. It affects the people around you and the success you have in all areas of your life. It's not just about losing a few pounds or a few inches. You never know the lives you're affecting when you do things to better your own body and health. I can't wait for you to make changes in your body and your life.

HOW TO HEAL WITH SUPERMARKET FOODS

Have you heard that the best things in life are free?

Well, I've found that some of the best things in life are at your local grocery store. When we did the research to understand what cured Brooke's lupus, we were shocked, amazed, and delighted to find that all the ingredients and the medicine that's necessary to cure not just lupus, but any inflammatory disease, is right at your local grocery store. This means it is accessible by *anybody*, anywhere, at any time, for a very low price. In this section, I'm going to teach you how to eat in a way that can reverse just about any inflammatory disease, including lupus, 100 percent.

The Lupus Cure Research

The first thing Brooke and I looked at was the diet I had put on her on that seemed to cure her lupus.

What was it about that diet that healed her disease?

The diet had a few key components:

- It was extremely high in raw vegetables.
- It was extremely high in omega-3 fatty acids.
- It included a large amount of water.

We started to research why raw vegetables and produce — especially green and cruciferous vegetables — have such a positive effect on one's health. One thing we kept seeing over and over in our research was that those particular foods are extremely anti-inflammatory; when you eat these foods, they have an amazing effect on dramatically lowering inflammation.

Brooke was eating tons of raw vegetables — more than twelve cups of raw vegetables every single day. When we measured the anti-inflammatory effects, they were through the roof. What she was eating was reducing all the inflammation in her body. Since lupus is an inflammatory disease, we were making it impossible for the lupus to stay present in her body.

Second, the diet was extremely high in omega-3 fatty acids. Sources of omega-3s are:

- Flaxseeds
- Chia seeds
- Flaxseed oil
- Chia seed oil

At the time, she was using fish oil to get her omega-3s; since then, we've found better sources. What we learned is that omega-3s are also one of the most powerful anti-inflammatory foods you can eat. We learned later that they're responsible not only for reducing inflammation, but they're also the building blocks of the cell walls. The health of the cell walls determines how efficiently and effectively your cells receive the chemical information in your body to help improve your metabolism and improve your health. Her cells were not very healthy; they weren't receiving the healing signals from the immune system effectively. They were sick, so the omega-3s were not only helping reduce inflammation, but were also improving the strength and effectiveness of her body's healing mechanisms.

Finally, the third component was lots and lots of water. What we found out later, through research, is that water is the medium by which almost every chemical process in the body occurs. If there's not enough water in the body, healing processes can't occur effectively. It's also the transport medium to flush out toxins from the body. Those toxins, if they stay in the body, can make the body sick, and the water helps transport them out of the body.

Basically, what I was using to help people lose weight and improve their health was also ideal for reducing inflammation, flushing out toxins, and allowing the body to heal, which was what helped Brooke cure her lupus. And exercise shuttles nutrients to every part and region of your body, because your heart pumps faster and harder, allowing the nutrients in the bloodstream to get to places where they usually can't if you're sedentary and not very active. So exercise, combined with a highly anti-inflammatory diet, were the keys to Brooke's cure of an incurable disease, and how quickly she was able to do it.

The Three Healing Ingredients

Let's go over these three healing ingredients you can find at your grocery store.

1. Produce—raw, living vegetables. The reason I'm saying vegetables and not fruits is because vegetables have an extremely high nutrient density compared to all other types of produce. When you go to the grocery store, I want you to buy as many raw vegetables as you possibly can, because they have the highest density of minerals, vitamins, and fiber out of all the foods you could possibly eat.

When the vegetables are raw and fresh, they have also the highest density of phytonutrients and enzymes, which:

- Improve your health
- Make food easily digestible
- Help you better utilize all the amazing nutrients in your body
- Raise your metabolism

I want you to enjoy as much raw food as you possibly can. The best part about it is the more you eat, the greater you increase your health, and the more weight you lose, too.

2. Get your omega-3s. The best sources of omega-3s come from plants; chia seeds and flaxseeds are two of the highest sources of omega-3s in the plant world. It is important that when you purchase these ingredients they are not roasted, cooked, or heated in any way, because omega-3s are very delicate; they break down when enough heat is applied to them. So get your omega-3s from raw chia seeds or flaxseeds. Or, if it's more convenient, you can purchase flaxseed oil or chia seed oil. You'll always find them in the refrigerated section of the health store or the health food department of your local grocery store.

3. Water. Make sure you drink at least ninety-six ounces or more of water a day. It's easy. You'll end up peeing a little bit more, but it's worth the health and the vitality you're going to get by releasing all those toxins from your body.

Summary

Make sure that at least 60 percent of everything you eat, your entire diet, is from wonderful, raw vegetables. If you're suffering from a disease right now, then you want to try to make sure at least 90 percent of your diet comes from those raw vegetables. The more you get in, the faster you will heal.

Second, make sure that you consume at least a handful of chia seeds or flaxseeds a day. If you decide that you'd prefer the concentrated oils, get at least a tablespoon of either chia seed oil or flaxseed oil. You can do one or the other or a combination. If you're suffering from a disease, then feel free to have more. The more, the better — have several tablespoons or several handfuls a day. Finally, make sure you get at least ninety-six ounces of water a day. If you're suffering from a disease, then I recommend you drink at least a gallon of water every day.

Often, when clients first start my programs, they ask about the latest supplements and workout fads on TV. The reality is that many of those are just designed to sell a product. The real answers are at the grocery store, and the real reason you don't find products or systems designed around grocery store food is because there's not big money to be made.

There's no money in selling grocery store foods, compared to making money by convincing people that they need to take a certain pill or a supplement each day or month. There's no money to be made in me telling you that you can get ten to one hundred times better results by simply going to your grocery store and buying the foods that are available right there, every single day.

Neither is there any money in telling you to simply exercise using your body weight, or joining a gym and learning how to use the equipment there, when other companies can try to convince you that you need a certain device to be able to do special exercises or to work out.

My intent is to get you results. That's always been my job. I practice one religion, and that's the religion of results. When you follow the information I am giving you in this book, you will get sensational results, faster than you ever dreamed possible.

CHAPTER THREE

Fat Loss Made Fast and Easy

FAT-LOSS NUTRITION

There's a lot of information out there on the best ways to lose fat and lose weight, and I've studied many of them. They mostly say the same thing:

- Reduce calories
- Reduce dietary fat
- Reduce carbohydrates

But that's not really the best way to do it. What happens when you reduce your food intake is you're slowing your metabolism. The way you want to lose fat is a better, smarter way. You want to reduce fat in a way that raises or maintains your metabolism, while putting your body in a biological state so that it is ready to lose all the fat you want.

Characteristics of a Fat-Loss Diet

The characteristics of a fat-loss diet that raises metabolism and helps you lose all the fat you want has three components:

- High nutrient intake
- Enough omega-3s
- High water intake

A high-nutrient intake comes from consuming a lot of fresh, raw vegetables. You can't beat the combination of the nutrients, phytonutrients, minerals, and vitamins that are in raw vegetables with low sugar content. Vegetables are, by far, the very best source of carbohydrates for anyone who wants to raise their metabolism and lose body fat. The benefits of fresh, raw vegetables include:

- They're delicious.
- They're absolutely nourishing.
- They raise your metabolism.
- They fill you up really fast.

The best part is you can eat an unlimited number of raw vegetables and not only will you not gain fat, you will accelerate your fat loss.

The second component is making sure that you're getting enough omega-3s. Flaxseeds and chia seeds are the best sources of plant-based omega-3s available. Omega-3s raise your metabolism. And, even though it's counterintuitive, they help you *lose* fat even though they're a form of fat, because they are the actual raw materials for the walls of every cell in your body, including fat and muscle cells. The more omega-3s you consume, the better all your cells that are involved with fat loss will function. In other words, you are providing more of the materials that your body needs to be able to lose more fat. When you increase your intake of omega-3s, you increase how much fat you can lose.

The third component of a fat-loss diet is high water intake. The best results I have seen for fat-loss is at least ninety-six ounces of water per day. That's three quarters of a gallon of water. I know that sounds like a lot, but it's absolutely worth it when you think of all the benefits you're going to get when you drink a lot of water:

- Almost every chemical process in the human body works via the medium of water; if you don't have enough water, you're going to shut down certain processes, and many of them are involved with fat loss.

- Adequate water keeps extra carbohydrates from being stored as body fat, and means they can be stored as something called *muscle glycogen*, which is the stored form of carbohydrates in muscles.

- Water makes a big difference in flushing out toxins from the body.

- The more water you consume, the healthier you're going to be and the more weight you're going to lose.

Fast-Metabolism Meals

Fast-metabolism meals are one of the easiest and quickest ways to create your nutrition program, because they follow the rules of maintaining a fast metabolism, without adding foods that cause you to gain fat. Make sure that each of your fast-metabolism meals contains about 75 percent of raw vegetables—whole, raw, high nutrient-dense vegetables. The extra 25 percent should contain a combination of fruits and omega-3 sources like chia seeds and flaxseeds. If you do that, ideally, for every one of your meals, and combine it with the proper exercise, you will accelerate your fat loss and set your body up so it can lose the maximum amount of fat.

Fat-Loss Meal Recipes

If you haven't noticed, the template for creating a fast-metabolism meal is identical to the template for making a fast-metabolism smoothie. You can replace any fast-metabolism meal with a fast-metabolism smoothie. A fast-metabolism smoothie *is* a fast-metabolism meal.

If you are like many of my students, a few times a day you *need* to have meals that you can chew. The only objection I ever hear about these great fat-loss meals is that many people complain about not having a lot of time to make their own food. If that's your situation, don't worry.

To make your life much easier, here are four of my favorite fat-loss, high-metabolism meal recipes that you can create in just minutes, with just a few ingredients, and a few tools in the kitchen.

Steamed Kale Tofu

> 16 oz. kale, pre-washed, pre-cut
> 14 oz. block of tofu
> ¼ cup nutritional yeast
> 14 oz. mushrooms, fresh
> 1 avocado
> 3 tbsp. Bragg Liquid Aminos

Empty the entire bag of kale, the entire block of tofu (cut up), and a large handful of mushrooms into a large pot. Add enough water for steaming. Steam on high for about 3 minutes with the lid on. Pour out the water, sprinkle on nutritional yeast, Bragg Liquid Aminos for flavor, and some cut-up avocado for an incredibly delicious fat-loss meal loaded with nutrients.

Steamed Spinach Tempeh

16 oz. pre-washed spinach
14 oz. block of tempeh
¼ cup nutritional yeast
1 onion, sliced
14 oz. mushrooms, fresh
3 tbsp. Bragg Liquid Aminos

Empty the entire bag of spinach, the entire block of tempeh (broken up), sliced onion, and mushrooms into a large pot for steaming. Spray Bragg Liquid Aminos on everything inside. Add enough water in the pot for steaming. Then steam on high for 3 minutes. Drain, sprinkle on nutritional yeast for flavor, and you are ready to enjoy another nutrient-rich, fat-loss meal.

Kale Edamame Salad

16 oz. kale, pre-washed, pre-cut
14 oz. shelled soybeans
1 cup red peppers, diced
1 cup tomato, diced
¼ cup nutritional yeast
¼ vegan salad dressing

Put the kale, soybeans, red peppers, and tomato into a salad bowl and mix it all up. Then pour on the vegan salad dressing. Yes, it's that easy!

Field Greens Tempeh Salad

16 oz. field greens, pre-washed
14 oz. block of tempeh
1 cup red peppers, diced
1 cup tomato, diced
¼ cup nutritional yeast
¼ cup vegan dressing

Break up the tempeh into small, bite-sized chunks and place in a baking pan. Sprinkle nutritional yeast on it and bake or toast it for 10 minutes at 450 degrees. Pour the prepared tempeh into a mixing bowl with all the other ingredients and mix it up. Pour on the vegan salad dressing and you are done.

Creating Your Fat-Loss Meal Plan

One of the biggest keys to success with my clients has been meal planning. In the beginning, most people are not used to eating the way I have been describing, so it's very important that you plan your meals ahead of time. I'm going to show you a system to make this really easy. One thing I've found is that convenience trumps all, so my recommendation is to either end every evening or start every day by making two or three fast-metabolism smoothies. Just throw some ingredients in a blender, turn it on for two to three minutes, pour it into jars, and you've already got half your meals made for the day.

The other strategy is to make your favorite fast-metabolism meals in bulk, all at once. Get at least three to five containers, and make your favorite meals in bulk. Choose one or two recipes that you enjoy and make two to three servings at one time, put them in storage containers, and keep them in the fridge. Every time you're hungry for a meal, which could be anywhere between two and five hours, just reach into the fridge and you've got a fast-metabolism meal or smoothie ready to go. You can take them to work, to the gym for after your workout, and when traveling. You'll have easy, delicious, fast-metabolism meals ready to go, and that will help you lose a lot of fat very quickly.

Notice that we are not concerned with calories as a tool for creating body transformation and weight loss. I find counting calories to be ineffective. I've worked with many clients, and I've used the caloric model. I was always scratching my head, wondering why simply reducing calories didn't work for everybody. That's when I realized that calories are simply a unit of heat and a unit of energy, not a predictor of how good your body is going to look and feel.

When you make the incorrect assumption that every bite of food you eat is either going to be used for energy or stored as energy for later, you are going to be very disappointed in your results.

Some of the foods you eat will be used, and maybe stored, as energy, but the rest of it will be used for other functions such as providing the raw material to create tissue, hormones, and neurotransmitters.

All the food you eat is not burned up as fat. Our bodies preferentially use carbohydrates as a form of fuel. Calories become a very ineffective tool for understanding how to achieve weight loss. Instead, we look at nutrients. We look at feeding our body what it needs so that it can lose fat. The way we tell our body to lose fat is through exercise.

Many people make the mistake of trying to lose weight by going on a low-calorie diet, which does not supply their bodies with enough of the nutrients that they need. Then they try to tell their body to lose weight by exercising, but their body doesn't lose the weight because it doesn't have the right materials needed to perform all the functions needed to optimize fat loss. So we're going to take a better approach: we're going to give the body everything it needs, and then we're going to tell it to lose weight by performing fat-loss exercises.

FAT-LOSS EXERCISE

In almost every single nutrition and diet book I've ever read, diet has always been the number-one thing everybody says you're going to need to concentrate on to lose weight.

They say, "Diet is 90 percent."

And I disagree 100 percent. I think diet accounts for 50 percent, at best, and here's why: I have known many people who can do tons of exercise, and they lose weight. It might not be a lot, but they're able to lose the weight. You can brute force your way through weight loss, if you want to. I've known athletes with the most horrible, high-calorie, junk-food diets who stay lean by doing three to four hours of intense exercise a day. It's absolutely possible to be able to lose weight with a bad diet.

However, if you're trying to lose weight just through diet—100 percent through diet—what that means is you're going to achieve a lower weight by losing fat AND muscle. Your body's going to start leeching from itself to get the nutrients it needs. Starvation is not the key. Instead, what you want is to provide your body with all the nourishment it needs so that all your body's cells can do their jobs. One of those jobs that your body can do is to lose weight. We're going to use the language of exercise to tell the body to lose as much weight from fat as humanly possible.

Characteristics of Fat-Loss Exercise

A long time ago, I was hired by a company called Star Trac to create the weight loss programs for the fitness equipment line featured on the hit TV show, *The Biggest Loser*. Through that experience, I worked with some of the top fat-loss experts in the world, and I learned a lot. I want to share those gems with you so you can start losing fat right away.

When it comes to exercise, it's very important that you understand all the aspects of exercise that can help you lose the greatest amount of fat. One, when you're choosing an exercise, you want to choose exercises that burn the greatest amount of calories in the least amount of time, because you want every minute that you spend working out in the gym, or at home, as productive as possible to reduce the fat from your body. That requires high-calorie burn.

How do you burn a lot of calories?

Here's the secret: involve as much muscle as you possibly can. This does not necessarily mean lifting weights, although I will show you how to lift weights to lose a lot of fat and burn a lot of calories. The idea is to get as much of your body involved as you possibly can. Many people go to the gym and work out their arms, then their legs, isolating their muscles one at a time. The sad part is, although they strengthen those muscles, they're not burning a lot of calories. That's why people don't see very fast results when they exercise that way.

You want to choose exercises that use as much muscle as possible. There are two methods for that:

- High-intensity interval training
- Functional resistance training

The more muscle you engage and activate during a workout, the greater the number of calories burned. The way you know you're burning a lot of calories is by your heart rate. The harder and faster your heart is beating, the more your muscles are demanding oxygen. Your heart only beats fast when more oxygen is being demanded. That means you are activating more muscle, because the more you activate muscle, the more oxygen your body needs. Your heart rate is your speedometer for how many calories you're burning. Let's discuss the main ways to burn a lot of fat.

High-Intensity Interval Training Cardio

Let's start with cardio.

Most people, when they think of losing weight and losing fat, think of doing cardio:

- Running or jogging

- Swimming
- Biking
- Walking
- Hiking

That's fine if you want to lose fat and weight the slow way. But if you want to do it faster, you're going to want to do what's called *high-intensity interval training cardio*. Studies have shown that when you do high-intensity interval training cardio, you burn up to nine times more body fat than you do in the same amount of time doing any other form of cardio.

What is high-intensity interval cardio?

It's simply this. You're still going to do a cardio workout; it could be any method you choose. But the intensity is split up into intervals. For example, you start off jogging for a few minutes, and then you'll launch into a high-intensity, all-out sprint for fifteen to forty-five seconds, as fast as you can — like a bear is chasing you in the woods — to the point where you're beyond exhausted. After the fifteen to forty-five seconds, which is what we call the *sprint interval*, you bring it down to a *recovery interval*, where you'll spend a little longer, between thirty and ninety seconds, doing what's called a *recovery pace*. You'll go back to the jogging pace. You're going to be out of breath, because you're recovering from the sprint interval that you just did. That's what the slower, or the lower intensity, jogging pace is for. After another thirty to ninety seconds of the jogging pace, you launch back into the sprint for another fifteen to forty-five seconds.

You go back and forth for the amount of time you are working out. I suggest a minimum of twenty minutes to a full hour. I promise you will notice a big difference in how much higher your heart will pump during your whole workout. You'll also notice a big difference in how much more sweat you generate doing that workout. If you do it on a regular basis — I recommend between three and five days a week — you will notice a *huge* difference in your weight loss and fat loss when you combine it with a fast-metabolism diet.

Resistance Training for Fat Loss

The second method for losing a lot of fat very quickly through exercise is by using functional resistance training exercises. These are exercises that use the *whole* body, including:

- Compound movements like Olympic lifts, squats, deadlifts, snatches, and cleans

- Exercises like floor-planks, push-ups, and different yoga poses

Below is a seven-day workout plan, complete with exercise descriptions, that you can do for a full week. They are designed to be done consecutively. You can perform them every day and then repeat for four to eight weeks. You can insert these workouts for any fat-loss day, (intervals of fat loss and muscle building are explained later).

Perform each exercise in a workout for forty-five to sixty seconds. How long you go depends on your level of fitness. Aim to rest as little as possible in between sets. Ten to thirty seconds of rest is a great goal that will produce enormous improvements in your cardiovascular system and fast fat loss. After your short rest, move on to the next exercise.

Performing one exercise, then another, and then another is called circuit training. They can be performed in any order. Sometimes when performing two exercises that require two different pieces of equipment on opposite sides of the gym, it might not be feasible to circuit them together, because of the long walk it takes to get from one to the other. In those cases, feel free to create sub-circuits.

In other words, if a workout has six different exercises, you can spend thirty minutes circuiting between the first three exercises, because the equipment needed for those exercises is close by. Then, you can spend thirty minutes circuiting between the last three exercises. You can mix them up any way you choose.

Perform as many rounds in a circuit as you wish. A common goal I try to achieve for my clients is thirty to sixty minutes total for each workout.

Some exercises will require weight equipment, while others will be based on your own body weight. If you are using weight equipment, select your weight in a way that will make you completely exhausted by forty-five to sixty seconds. The number of repetitions does not matter. You can do them fast or slow. The time you spend performing each exercise is what matters.

We call this *time under tension*. If you are doing a body weight exercise, adjust your speed so that you go to full exhaustion within forty-five to sixty seconds. If an exercise is unilateral, meaning you do one side at a time, then you perform one side of the exercise for forty-five to sixty seconds and then the other side for the same amount of time.

Day 1

Exercise: Floor Alternating Knee-Ins

Preparation:

> Assume push-up position on hands and toes.
>
> Keep hips in neutral position with back straight, preventing the pelvis from dipping or peaking.

Movement:

> Swing one leg out and bend the knee, trying to touch the elbow on the same side.
>
> Hold and then bring leg back to starting position and repeat with opposite side.
>
> Avoid letting back dip down during movement.

Exercise: Bidirectional Cable Rotations

Equipment: dual adjustable pulley

Preparation:

> Adjust cable height to the level of your chest.
>
> Stand facing toward the cable pulley with the handle aligned with the middle of your body.
>
> Grab handle and create tension by taking two steps back.

With feet shoulder-width apart, squat down until the pulley is even with your shoulders.

Movement:

With arms remaining outstretched, twist at the waist to one side until shoulders face opposite wall.

Hold and then twist 180 degrees past the starting point in opposite direction.

Hold and repeat movement.

Exercise: Frontal Squat to Push Press

Equipment: dumbbells

Preparation:

Stand with feet shoulder-width apart with a dumbbell in each hand.

Raise dumbbells to ear level with palms facing outward.

Movement:

Step out to one side and squat down while lowering dumbbells to ear level.

Hold and then return to standing position with weights pressed overhead and palms facing outward.

Hold and then repeat.

Exercise: Ball Crunches

Equipment: fitness ball

Preparation:

> Lie across exercise ball with both feet on the ground and torso raised parallel to the floor.
>
> Cross both arms across your chest, making sure you are outstretched over the ball.

Movement:

> Start in the outstretched position and curl abdomen upward to a 45-degree angle.
>
> Hold and then slowly recline back and stretch back out over the ball and repeat movement.

Exercise: Squat to Bilateral Row

Equipment: dual adjustable pulley

Preparation:

> Adjust cable height to the level of your chest.
>
> Stand facing toward the cable pulley with the handle aligned with the middle of your body.

Grab handles with each hand and create tension by taking two steps back.

With feet shoulder-width apart, squat until the pulley is even with your shoulders.

Movement:

Squat with arms outstretched and pause.

With your elbows at your sides, return to standing while simultaneously bringing the handles to your stomach.

Hold and then return to squatting position with arms fully extended in front of you.

Exercise: Lunge Walk With Alternating Arm Bicep Curl

Equipment: dumbbells

Preparation:

Stand with dumbbells in each hand in an open area.

Keep your elbows plugged into your sides during the entire exercise.

Movement:

Step out as far as possible and lower back knee to just above the ground.

While you are lunging, slowly curl with the opposite arm so that your arm makes a *V*.

Hold at the bottom of the lunge, then return to standing position while extending curled arm.

Immediately lunge forward with your other leg and repeat the same lunge-and-curl motion.

Day 2

Exercise: Side Plank

Preparation:

Start by lying on your side, legs straight, feet stacked.

Straighten bottom arm, keeping it in line below shoulder, and place free hand on your hip.

Flex feet and balance on sides of feet (feet are stacked).

Movement:

Lift hips off the ground while keeping your body from bending and hold the position.

Exercise: Seated Cable Row

Equipment: dual adjustable pulley

Preparation:

> Sit on the bench with both feet planted on the platform.

> Keep knees slightly bent and your back straight.

Movement:

> Draw your abdomen inward toward the spine.

> Row the bar by flexing your elbows and bringing the thumbs toward your armpits while retracting and depressing your shoulder blades.

> Avoid letting your back arch with your head jutting forward.

> Hold and then slowly return the arms to original position by extending the elbows.

Exercise: Ball Knee-In

Equipment: fitness ball

Preparation:

> Place both elbows on exercise ball, keeping them in line with your shoulders.

> Rise onto your toes into a push-up position, keeping your back and legs straight.

Movement:

> Hold extended position while balancing on the ball, making sure to keep your back straight.

Exercise: One-Arm Low Row

Equipment: dual adjustable pulley

Preparation:

> Adjust cable height to the lowest setting toward the ground.

> Stand facing toward the cable pulley with the handle aligned with the arm you are pulling with.

> Grab handle and create tension by taking two steps back.

> Place feet shoulder-width apart.

Movement:

> Squat with your arm outstretched and your glutes pushed out.

> Stand up from the squat while simultaneously pulling the handle to your side.

> Hold and repeat squat-and-row movement.

Day 3

Exercise: One-Arm Curl With Split Stance

Equipment: dual adjustable pulley

Preparation:

> Stagger feet with one foot in front of you and one in back with a slight bend in both knees.

> Adjust the pulley to just above your shoulder and grip handle with your arm outstretched and parallel to the ground.

Movement:

> While keeping your arm parallel to the ground, curl weight toward your forehead.

> Hold and return to starting position.

Exercise: Ball Supine Tricep Extension

Equipment: fitness ball, dumbbells

Preparation:

> Lie on the ball with it supporting your shoulders, head, and neck only.

> Keep your back straight during the entire movement.

Bring dumbbells up and in line with your shoulders.

Movement:

While keeping your arms perpendicular to the ground, lower the weight toward your forehead.

Hold and then extend your arms back up to the starting position.

Exercise: One-Arm Tricep Extensions Facing Away

Equipment: dual adjustable pulley

Preparation:

Adjust cable pulley to above your shoulder.

Grab handle, take two big steps forward, and stand facing away from the pulley.

Make sure your arm is parallel to the floor.

Movement:

With your knees slightly bent and your arm still parallel to the floor, extend your arm out away from your body.

Hold and then return to starting position.

Exercise: Two-Arm Squat Curl

Equipment: dumbbells

Preparation:

> Stand with your feet shoulder-width apart, your back straight, and dumbbells in each hand.

Exercise:

> Slowly squat, making sure to jut out your hips, and let the weight hang at your sides.

> Hold, then stand up slowly while simultaneously curling both weights about 80 percent of the way up.

> Hold and then return the weights to your sides while squatting down for the next repetition.

Day 4

Exercise: Ball Hamstring Curls

Equipment: dumbbells

Preparation:

> Lie on the ground with your legs resting on the exercise ball.

Only your ankles should be making contact with the top of the ball.

Raise your hips up off the ground with your hands out to your sides for balance.

Movement:

Curl your legs underneath you, as if you are trying to touch your heels to your rear end.

Hold and then slowly extend your legs back out to the starting position.

Exercise: One-Arm Military Press With Lunge

Equipment: dumbbells

Preparation:

Stand with your feet shoulder-width apart and with a dumbbell raised to ear level (your palm facing out).

Movement:

Lunge forward and with your opposite arm, press up with the dumbbell, extending your arm fully.

Hold and then return to standing while lowering the weight down to ear level.

Hold and then repeat motion.

Exercise: Squat Jumps With Stabilization

Preparation:

Stand with your feet shoulder-width apart and your toes slightly turned out.

Movement:

Slowly squat down, making sure to keep your knees behind your toes.

Jump up as high as you can, trying to touch the ceiling.

Land softly on the balls of your feet while immediately beginning to squat into next repetition.

Exercise: One-Arm Upright Row With Squat

Equipment: dual adjustable pulley

Preparation:

Adjust pulley height to lowest setting.

Stand with the pulley in the center of your stance, your feet wider than shoulder-width apart.

Grip the handle and flex your core.

Movement:

Squat down with your rear end out and your arm outstretched.

Hold, then as you stand up, raise your elbow up and bring your hand all the way to your cheek.

Hold at the top and repeat.

Day 5

Exercise: Straight Bar Chest Press

Equipment: dual adjustable pulley

Preparation:

Stand behind bar, facing away from the cable pulley system.

Space your hands wider than shoulder-width apart on the bar.

Take two or three steps forward and away from system to create tension.

Stagger your feet, placing one foot forward and one behind.

Movement:

> While keeping your arms parallel to the floor, press weight away from your body.

> Hold and then slowly return weight to your chest.

Exercise: Two-Arm Dumbbell Stationary Lunge

Equipment: dumbbells

Preparation:

> Stand with your feet staggered with one in front and one in back, with a dumbbell in each hand.

> Flex your core before beginning exercise, and hold it flexed throughout the exercise.

Movement:

> Slowly lower down into a lunge position, hovering your back knee just above the ground.

> Hold and then slowly extend back up until you return to your starting position.

Exercise: Push-Ups

Preparation:

> Place your hands wider than shoulder-width apart on the ground, making sure your wrists are over your elbows.

Keep your back straight and in neutral position with your feet together and your head up.

Movement:

While keeping your entire body straight, bend your elbows and lower your chest to just a few inches above the ground.

Hold and then push up to your starting position.

Exercise: Burpees (No Weights)

Preparation:

Stand in an open area with plenty of space behind you.

Movement:

Bend your knees and place both hands on the ground.

Kick both legs out behind you and assume a push-up position.

Hold then bring both feet back to your hands and jump up into the air.

Land softly and repeat movement.

Exercise: Squats

Equipment: smith machine or Max Rack

Preparation:

>Place bar just below shoulder height on rack before loading weight onto either side.

>Prior to beginning squat, make sure the bar is resting off the neck and on your shoulders.

>Space feet shoulder-width apart with your weight mainly on your heels.

Movement:

>Bend both knees and squat down, making sure to jut out hips and rear.

>If possible, lower to where your legs are parallel with the floor and your back is straight.

>Hold, then drive upward to starting position.

Day 6

Exercise: Ball Walk-Outs

Equipment: fitness ball

Preparation:

>Make sure you are in an open area with plenty of space in front of you.

>Lie over exercise ball, facing the ground.

Movement:

> Roll forward on the ball until both hands are touching the ground.
>
> Walk your hands out while balancing your legs on the ball; move out as far as you can while keeping your back straight.
>
> Hold and then slowly walk back in toward the starting position.

Exercise: Unidirectional Cable Wood Chops

Equipment: dual adjustable pulley

Preparation:

> Adjust cable height to the highest position.
>
> Stand facing perpendicular to the cable pulley.
>
> Grab handle and create tension by taking two steps back.
>
> Stand with feet shoulder-width apart and knees slightly bent.

Movement:

> Keeping your arms straight, twist your torso, bringing your hands down to your opposite ankle.

Hold and slowly return to the starting position.

Exercise: Ball Push-Ups

Equipment: fitness ball

Preparation:

> Place your hands on an exercise ball, making sure your wrists are over your elbows.
>
> Keep your back straight and in neutral position with your feet together and your head up.

Movement:

> While keeping your entire body straight, bend your elbows and lower your chest to just a few inches above the ball.
>
> Squeeze and hold, then push up to your starting position.

Exercise: Squat to One-Arm Row

Equipment: dual adjustable pulley

Preparation:

> Adjust cable height to be even with your chest.
>
> Stand facing toward the cable pulley with the handle aligned with the arm you are pulling with.

Grab handle and create tension by taking two steps back.

Place feet shoulder-width apart.

Movement:

Squat down with your arm outstretched and your glutes pushed out.

Stand up from the squat while simultaneously pulling the handle to your side.

Hold and repeat the squat-and-row movement.

Day 7

Exercise: Floor Oblique Suitcase Crunch

Preparation:

Lay on your side with your hips jutting out.

Place your top arm up and over your head, stretching out your side.

Movement:

With a quick, explosive movement, crunch up and try to touch your toes with your top hand, making yourself into a *V* shape.

Hold and then slowly return back to starting position, remaining on your side.

Exercise: Back Lunge to Tricep Pushdown

Equipment: dual adjustable pulley

Preparation:

Adjust cable height to the highest position.

Stand facing toward the cable.

Grab ropes with both hands and keep arms at your sides.

Stand with feet shoulder-width apart and knees slightly bent.

Movement:

Step backward with one foot as far as possible.

Bend your knees, bringing you down toward the ground.

Simultaneously extend both hands down, keeping your arms at your sides.

Hold lunge and tricep extension.

Step back up and bend arms back to 45-degree angle.

Hold and repeat.

Exercise: Unidirectional Cable PNF (Proprioceptive Neuromuscular Facilitation)

Equipment: dual adjustable pulley

Preparation:

> Adjust cable height to the lowest position.
>
> Stand facing perpendicular to the cable pulley.
>
> Grab handle and create tension by taking two steps back.
>
> Stand with feet shoulder-width apart and knees slightly bent.

Movement:

> Keeping your arms straight, twist your torso, bringing your hands up and over your opposite shoulder.
>
> Hold and slowly return to the starting position.

Exercise: One-Leg Barbell Curl

Equipment: barbell

Preparation:

> Stand, gripping the barbell with feet and hands shoulder-width apart.
>
> Contract your core muscles and raise one leg.

Movement:

> With your core flexed and your elbows at your side, curl weight 80 percent of the way up.

> Hold and return weight to starting position.

The key to these exercises, and why they work so well, is that they use the whole body; they use a huge amount of muscle tissue. Instead of counting repetitions, what's important when doing resistance exercise for fat loss is the amount of time you're spending, forcing your muscles to be under tension. When muscles are under tension, they're burning calories.

When your muscles are relaxed or not under tension, they're not doing much for you at all. *You want to spend forty-five to sixty seconds performing each exercise.* That means that you've got a lot of muscle tissue under tension. This produces the best results possible for fat loss: minimizing your rest and *taking ten to thirty seconds between sets before moving onto the next exercise.* Also it's a great opportunity for you to link four or five exercises into a circuit, in which you do one exercise after the next.

Again, it's about making your muscles work as much as they can, and getting as many of the muscles to work as hard as they can for the longest amount of time. Often, when people go to the gym, they do a set — which lasts for about eighteen seconds — and then get a drink of water, and come back to do their next set after one or two minutes, which means they're only working out for six to twelve minutes during an entire one hour workout.

If you work out in the way I've outlined, you're forcing your muscles to work for thirty to forty-five minutes instead. That's anywhere from three to six times what most people do when they go the gym. And instead of working out one muscle group, you're working out multiple muscle groups, which doubles, triples, even quadruples the amount of calorie burn that you're getting in the same amount of time. That is the key to losing a lot of fat quickly.

Creating Your Fat-Loss Workout Routine

Planning your workouts is also another key to success. Just like your diet, you want to plan your workouts as well, so they are easy and enjoyable. You want to plan your workouts so that they consistently fit your schedule. You can go to the gym and do one of these wonderful workouts once or twice, but unfortunately, it's going to take a lot more than that. If you let too much time pass before your next workout, chances are you're not going to see the results you want. You want to be consistent. Make sure it's part of your schedule.

When you're trying to lose as much fat as possible, I recommend allocating an hour a day, between four and six days of the week—even seven if you're able to—for fat-loss exercises. When you do that, you will see amazing results. I've had clients who really wanted to see results fast, and they performed fat-loss exercises up to ninety minutes a day, six to seven days a week, and when they combined that with a fast-metabolism diet, they achieved results of seven pounds of weight loss in a single week, or dropping two to three dress sizes in three to four weeks. It's completely doable, and it's absolutely safe, but of course you want to do it at your level.

These clients obviously had the will, the determination, and the time to be able to do that. But if you don't have that much time, or that's hard for you to do, that's okay. If you can do four to six hours of fat-loss exercise per week, and if you stay committed to a fat-loss diet seven days a week, you are going to see amazingly dramatic results.

The best way to lose the greatest amount of fat is to use a combination of both high intensity interval training cardio and functional resistance training. Chances are, there are going to be days when your muscles are going to be very sore and it's going to be difficult for you to do another functional resistance training workout.

That's fine, because on those days, you can perform your high-intensity interval training cardio workout.

When you do cardio training, you aren't creating the same amount of strain in your muscles that you do when you perform resistance training. Most of the physical strain is put on your heart. While your skeletal muscles are taking a rest day, you can still work out your heart at a high intensity. This is important if you want to lose fat quickly, because sore muscles often keep people from working out.

Interval training cardio also has the tendency to decrease the time that it takes to recover from the weight-lifting workouts, because you're not putting a big strain on your muscles. In fact, what you're doing is improving the recovery by shuttling more blood and nutrients into those healing muscles. A great strategy is to alternate between high intensity interval training cardio and functional resistance training. Or, another way you can do it is by making half your workout high-intensity interval training cardio, and the other half functional resistance training for fat loss. Either way works. Try both and see what fits your personality and your body the best.

PUTTING IT INTO PRACTICE

Now you understand how to use fat-loss exercises to help you burn fat, lose weight, and get the body you want. Let's put it into practice. I'm going to share some of my best tips for manifesting the body of your dreams.

Fat-Loss Tools

There are certain tools that will make your life so much easier and will accelerate your results, if you use them.

These tools are optional, but I highly recommend that you get them:

- A stopwatch for high-intensity interval training cardio
- The *Fat Killer* mp3, available at SmoothieShred. com
- A seconds-counter app (free)
- Jump rope
- Resistance-training bands

When doing high-intensity interval training, you'll need to be able to time the intervals. My favorite intervals are between fifteen and forty-five seconds, and my favorite rest intervals are between thirty and ninety seconds. But unless you're keeping track of time, you're not going to be able to do your intervals effectively. That's where a stopwatch comes in handy.

Another tool I recommend is one I created, called *The Fat Killer*, an interval cardio trainer, in case you don't like carrying a stopwatch or having to check it. The Fat Killer is simply an mp3 that you download and put into your music player. If you're used to working out with earphones, it's very easy. All you do is press play, and I coach you through the sprint and recovery intervals, telling you when to sprint and when to breathe and recover, as well as mentally preparing you for an amazing workout. You can find it on my website, SmoothieShred.com.

If your stopwatch has a countdown timer, great. If not, I recommend you use an app on your smartphone. My favorite app for that is the "Seconds Timer," which you can find at the App Store. There is a free version and a paid version. The free version works just fine to help you manage your resistance training intervals.

Another tool I recommend is a jump rope. Jump ropes are affordable and a great way to be able to do your interval cardio. And it doesn't matter what the weather is outside; you can jump rope in a hallway of any hotel or inside your living room.

I also recommend resistance-training bands. They're inexpensive, and they are amazing for helping you do upper-body and lower-body exercises. They allow you to simulate health-club quality workouts. You can find these on my website, SmoothieShred.com.

Scheduling: Making the Time and Making It Happen

If you're not using a calendar program to schedule your day, I highly recommend that you do, especially a calendar with an alarm. If you use a paper calendar, that's fine, too. What's important is putting your workout time into your schedule. Always factor in the time it takes for you to get prepared and for any travel needed. That way, there's nothing that can get between you and your workout. If you're going to the gym, I recommend you add an extra ten minutes to get to the gym and get ready, and another ten minutes to get back, just in case.

Measuring Results

Whenever you are trying to lose weight and lose fat, you want to make sure you actually *are* losing weight and losing fat. You want to be measuring your results on a regular basis.

Three of my favorite ways to measure results are:

- Using a body weight scale
- Using a tape measure
- How well you're fitting into your clothes

There are three things that are going to happen when you lose body fat:

- Number one: you're going to lose weight. You're going to weigh less because you have less fat tissue on your body. You're carrying around less stuff on your body.

- Number two: you'll lose inches. A lot of the weight that you're going to lose is the fat around your belly. That's why you want to measure your waist, to see if it's getting smaller.

- Number three: you're also going to lose fat all over your body. Noticing how easily you're fitting in your clothes is another way to measure how well you are doing.

Now, when you're looking at the scale, understand that your weight is going to go up and down. This is normal, because your body weight is affected daily by hydration, food in your intestines, glycogen, and the last time you went to the bathroom. All those things will factor into your weight, but over time, if you are losing fat, you are permanently releasing tissue from your body.

What you're going to notice, through all the ups and downs, is if you're losing fat, your body weight will be trending downward. Measure the highs and lows on a week-to-week basis. After two to four weeks, if you're noticing the numbers decrease, then you are losing weight. When you notice that your waist measurement is getting smaller on a weekly basis, then you are losing weight from body fat. If you notice that your clothes are fitting better, then you are losing weight. Finally, taking before-and-after pictures is always a great way to see if you're getting smaller, losing fat, and getting leaner.

Case Studies

Gina

Gina hated her legs. She hated how big they had become, how they shook and jiggled every time she walked. Embarrassed and ashamed of her legs, she kept them hidden behind long skirts and long pants. The thought of wearing short skirts and short pants of any kind terrified her, and she hated the dressing-room mirror. And it was getting worse.

But it wasn't always that way.

Gina was in her mid-fifties when she noticed she had steadily gained weight year after year for the past ten years. Then menopause hit in her early fifties, and it got even worse. She went from a slender size 6 to well over a size 10.

She couldn't explain it. She hadn't changed her diet. She wasn't eating more, and she wasn't eating any differently.

Although she didn't exercise, she'd never had to in order to maintain the same size 6 she was since her early twenties.

Gina was always recognized by her friends and family as a woman with good genetics. She never seemed to gain weight; she was always thin. It turned out that her genetics were just as good as every one else's.

Her typical diet included a lot of carbohydrate-rich Polish and Jewish dishes that were made with a lot of potatoes, matzo, bread, and some cooked vegetables.

Water was rarely in her cup, as she drank mostly coffee and diet soda.

Her diet was virtually devoid of any living food nutrition and very low in whole food nutrition.

So how did she stay thin?

Her secret to staying thin was by eating very little. She ate one to two very small meals a day. Despite the low quality, high-fat food she ate, it wasn't enough to gain weight.

However, at times, when she ate too much she would gain weight very quickly, like everyone else. Only a few days of eating an extra dessert, eating too many pieces of rye bread, or enjoying too many pieces of New York pizza were all it took to gain an extra pound or two.

To combat this, she had a unique technique for losing the weight fast. She went on the *Diet Coke and sauerkraut diet*. That's right, she would drink nothing but Diet Coke and eat nothing but sauerkraut.

She rationalized that since the sauerkraut contained virtually no calories and the Diet Coke also had zero calories, she could eat and drink as much as she wanted to feel full, while taking in zero calories.

As odd as that diet may seem, it worked. She used it successfully every time she gained weight. After a few days or a few weeks of eating nothing but sauerkraut and drinking Diet Coke, she would lose any weight she had gained and was back to her slim and slender self.

However, her metabolism eventually paid a steep price. Like many hundreds of students who come to me for the first time, she believed that as you get older your metabolism naturally and uncontrollably gets slower.

The truth is that it's not your age that determines how fast your metabolism is. It's the number of consecutive years of high-quality nourishment that determines your metabolism.

In Gina's case, she spent twenty consecutive years starving the cells of her body and giving them the fewest and lowest-quality nutrients to function.

Let's take a look at the primary ingredients in Gina's diet. You might not be surprised that her metabolism kept her from achieving any significant results.

Gina was on the Nutrisystem program, which consisted of prepackaged meals made up of nothing but dead, processed food. Nothing she ate nourished her cells or helped her metabolism. Instead, it was doing the opposite. Her metabolism was getting worse, which easily explained why she gained weight and went up in size.

Gina spent a year investing up to eighty minutes in the gym Monday through Friday, with very little results to speak of. Working out on her own, combined with Nutrisystem, helped her lose a measly four pounds after an entire year.

That's when Gina became convinced that nothing but liposuction could help her lose the weight and regain her shape.

I offered Gina the opportunity to spend four weeks with me, allowing me to oversee her diet and exercise, and make recommendations as needed. I said if I couldn't help her lose at least four pounds of weight after four weeks with me, something was really wrong.

Gina accepted my offer and we got started.

First, I restructured her workout so she spent only forty-five minutes a day, four to five days a week, doing nothing but fat-loss exercises. I had her work to complete exhaustion with every exercise, and we minimized the amount of rest she took between sets. I also maximized the amount of muscle she was engaging with each workout. This drastically increased the number of calories she was burning with each workout.

Second, we got rid of Nutrisystem and added in the fast-metabolism meals. I had Gina eating five to six fast-metabolism meals per day — tons of vegetables, both raw and cooked, high omega-3s, lots of water, and lean protein.

After twenty-eight days, Gina had lost 12.2 pounds, three inches off her hips, three inches off her waist, and one-and-a-quarter inch off each thigh. She went from a size 10 pants to a junior size 7.

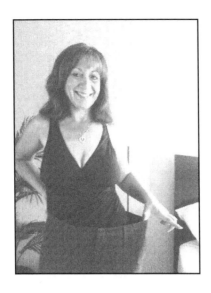

She was so thrilled at the results she achieved in just four weeks, she kept going. After ninety days she was down forty-two pounds and fitting comfortably into size 4 pants. This was the smallest size she'd ever worn in her entire adult life. In her 20s, she could only fit in a size 6. She was so happy with how flat and tight her stomach was, she had to get a belly-button ring.

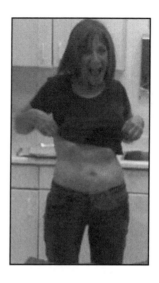

Gina's metabolism just would not quit. A year later, she is even leaner and fitter.

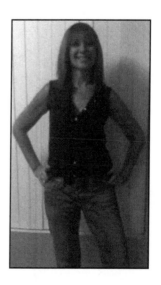

How I Saved My Dad's Life

I couldn't hold it in any longer; I got so pissed off at my dad that I blew up at him.

It was Christmas Eve, my oldest son, Solomon, was just two years old, and he loved his Grandpa so much. I took my family up to my parents' house to spend Christmas with them. It was always a happy time of year to be with my family, but this year was different.

Four weeks previously, my father sent the results of his blood sugar and lipid profile test to my wife to see if she had anything to say that his doctor hadn't already. My wife — a doctor, as I've mentioned before — has read hundreds of these reports and noticed a few alarming details.

"You're only two points away from full-blown diabetes!" exclaimed my wife. "Did you know that?"

My father looked confused. "My doctor said I was within normal range and didn't mention anything," he said.

According to my father's blood sugar test, he was just one bad meal away from getting full-blown diabetes. Diabetes would mean having to go on medication for the rest of his life and dying a slow, painful death.

Brooke explained this to my father, and he was in disbelief, wondering why his doctor didn't mention anything about it.

My father asked what he could do to reverse his pre-diabetic condition. So, we laid out a plan for him of what to eat and how to exercise.

The dietary guidelines were simple: eat a vegan diet, minimize processed foods, and exercise regularly. Stay away from all meat and dairy.

My father had been obese for as long as I could remember. He was never happy about his weight, but this was the first time it seemed to be a serious problem.

I remember my father trying many times to lose weight. His strategy was to skip breakfast, eat an apple for lunch, and have a light dinner at night. He would lose about twenty pounds over a few months and then slowly gain it all back. My poor dad starved on his diets; it was no wonder why he always gained the weight back. Starvation diet strategies never work in the long run. You simply get burned out on them.

My father committed to changing his diet. It seemed like Brooke's interpretation of his blood work scared him. This was the closest he had been to a devastating disease.

We arrived at my parents' house on Christmas Eve. Solomon immediately jumped out of the car and went to play with Grandpa. Grandpa was my son's best friend, and my father loved Solomon.

Soon, it was time for bed and everyone retired for the night.

The next morning, when we woke up, Solomon was playing in the living room, and my father was eating breakfast. I went over to see what healthy vegan option he had chosen to fight off the threat of diabetes.

What I saw him eating was a bowl of sugary Honey Smacks, filled to the top with cow's milk, and a big Costco blueberry muffin.

The only thought going through my head was what Brooke had said to him after she read his blood test results. "You're only two points away from full-blown diabetes!"

The very next sugary meal that my father ate could be the one that tipped his blood sugar over the edge into a full diagnosis of a terrible disease. One more bite of processed sugars, one more swig of cow's milk, or one more bite of processed carbohydrates could be all it took for him to become sick. And there he was, eating Sugar Smacks, drinking cow's milk, and munching on a muffin.

Tears began to well up in my eyes. I couldn't believe how irresponsible he was being with his health, especially after we had talked four weeks earlier.

I looked over at my son Solomon, who was quietly playing in the living room, and I couldn't take it anymore. I blew up.

I don't remember everything that I yelled at my dad, but I remember being overcome with emotion. My father refused to do anything different.

My mother yelled out, "You only live once!"

I thought to myself: *You only live once. Isn't that the truth?*

I couldn't stand to be in the house anymore, watching my father's health go down the tubes and listening to him defend his own limitations while my son was there.

That afternoon, we packed up our things and headed home. It was a quiet, hopeless drive.

A week went by before I received a phone call from my father. What he said shocked me.

"I'll follow your plan," he said.

I couldn't believe what he had just said. "Really? You're really going to follow our plan?"

"Yes, but I'm only going to do it for three months, and we'll see how it goes."

"I'll take anything you'll give me. I love you, Dad."

And thus began *Operation Save Dad*.

Saving my father was not going to be easy.

To reverse my father's pre-diabetic condition, fix his cholesterol, and help him lose the excess weight, I needed to design a workout and nutrition program to bring his blood sugar down while also keeping him full, nourished, and satisfied.

In the past, whenever my father had tried other diets, the feeling of hunger would be what took him down.

Knowing my father, I knew that it also needed to be simple. When it comes to diets and exercise, anything too complicated would go right over his head, and he wouldn't stick with it for long.

And the workouts needed to be easy enough for him to physically perform. My father was severely out of shape from never exercising.

Finally, the plan needed to achieve measurable results on a weekly basis.

Here's the plan I put my father on:

1. Drink at least three fast-metabolism smoothies per day, each time drinking until absolute fullness. His typical smoothie consisted of 90 percent Costco field greens or kale, and 10 percent flaxseeds and pineapple. The liquid was either water or almond milk.

2. Eat a high-vegetable dinner (cooked or raw), with no processed foods.

3. Twenty minutes per day of interval hill walking on treadmill, alternating one minute on a steep incline and one minute on no incline.

In the first three months, my father lost more than twenty pounds. He said he felt full all day and was completely satisfied with the smoothies alone. There were many days when he just drank the smoothies.

He loved it so much that he stayed on the plan. Within six months, he got his blood work retested and his cholesterol was normal, his blood sugar was optimal, and he had lost more than forty pounds.

His doctor took him off all medications. Today, my father has continued to lose even more weight, down more than fifty pounds, and is still medication-free.

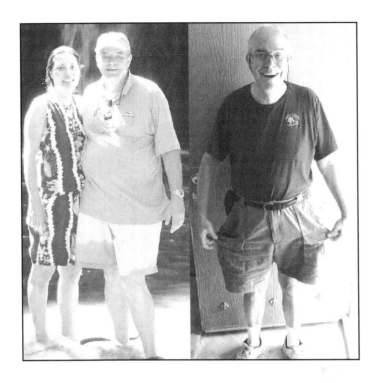

For hundreds of success stories, join our Smoothie Shred Facebook group at SmoothieShred.com.

When You've Decided You Want Help

Sometimes, as you're going through the process of body transformation, the results are not what you expect. The reason is you have no real reference to truly know what to expect, because there are so many different things going on in your body all at the same time. You just have to stick with the system and not do anything stupid.

If you notice you're not losing any weight after a week, it's okay. Give it another week, and if at that point you're still not losing weight, that's when it's time to seek help. Seeking help is one of the best things you can do, because there's a good chance it's not that the system isn't working for you, but that you're probably not working the system the way it was intended. There's probably something that you're doing wrong, so please don't be afraid to ask for help.

If you need help, please contact us. Go to Smoothie-Shred.com, and feel free to go to the contact page, and ask for the help you need. We are here for you, and we'll be happy to give you assistance and guide you in the right direction.

CHAPTER FOUR

Building Muscle Quickly at Any Age

MUSCLE-BUILDING NUTRITION

The other half of the coin when it comes to body transformation is building muscle. It's great to be able to lose fat, get more definition, and be leaner, but it's even better to be stronger, fitter, and have some nice muscles to show for it.

One of the hardest problems many people have when trying to get in better shape is losing fat while building muscle.

How do you lose fat and build muscle at the same time?

I know people who are good at losing body fat, but not so good at gaining muscle. I also know people who are great at gaining muscle and not so good at losing fat. Hopefully the last section solved a lot of the problems for anybody who has trouble losing fat.

This section explains how to make it easier to build muscle. This works for everyone, every time, and it's done in combination with a plant-based diet.

Characteristics of a Muscle-Building Diet

When building muscle, you need to provide your body with more raw materials in order for it to create more tissue than it has right now. One of the biggest mistakes that people make when trying to build muscle is they do muscle-building exercises and workouts, but because they want to stay lean, they don't eat enough food and nutrients to be able to build that extra muscle. So, their body doesn't change much.

Building muscle requires everything in surplus to create a surplus of tissue:

- More protein
- More carbohydrates
- More water
- More vitamins
- More minerals
- More fats

When putting together your muscle-building nutrition plan, you're going to start with the foundation of a fast-metabolism meal. Then you're going to add carbohydrates—good carbohydrates—on top of that. I recommend that you eat at least a handful of the carbohydrates of your choice in addition to your fast-metabolism meal. Good carbohydrates will form the energy and carbohydrate foundation for building lots of muscle. Your carbohydrates can be in the form of:

- Grains, such as rice
- Starches, such as potatoes
- Legumes, such as lentils

You're also going to add more protein. My favorite high-protein vegan foods for building muscle are:

- Tofu
- Tempeh
- Seitan
- Soybeans
- Vegan protein powders

These are the vegan protein powders I have used, from favorite to least favorite, with links to purchase them online:

- Warrior Force Elite Green Cool Green (amzn.to/1hYJ71a)

- PlantFusion Vanilla Bean (amzn.to/1k8bcEf)

- Sunwarrior Warrior Blend Vanilla and Chocolate (amzn.to/1fYt5Qw)

- Vega Sport Performance Protein Vanilla (amzn.to/1fikicl)

- Warrior Force Warrior Food Extreme Chocolate Plus (amzn.to/1dGaJHu)

- Pure Vegan Pea Protein Vanilla (amzn.to/MZxrQm)

You also want to increase your fats, both omega-3s and omega-6s.

Good sources of omega-3s are:

- Flaxseeds
- Chia seeds
- Flaxseed oil
- Chia seed oil

To get your omega-6s, you can eat:

- Any nuts in raw form
- Peanuts
- Almonds
- Cashews
- Macadamia nuts
- Seeds
- Walnuts

Make sure you are drinking a gallon of water a day, because you're going to need a lot of water to support all the new muscle you're building.

If you follow these guidelines with every single meal, and make sure you eat until uncomfortable fullness, you're going to do a good job setting your body up, so it can build a lot of muscle.

Right now your stomach is set to a certain size; you eat to fullness, then you naturally want to stop eating. That's because it's designed to keep you exactly the same size that you are. If you want to increase the size of your muscles, you are going to have to eat until uncomfortable fullness so your body gets the additional nutrients it needs. More nutrients are the key to being able to add more muscle and tissue.

Muscle-Building Meals

The two types of meals that I like to eat are smoothies and regular meals. Smoothies are great because they're:

- Convenient
- Easy to make
- Able to be prepared ahead of time
- Very portable
- Full of the nutrients you need

Anything that can go in a meal can go in a smoothie as well. Let's talk about how to build some of these meals. Let's start with a smoothie.

A muscle-building smoothie is a little different than a fast-metabolism smoothie. You're going to consume both. I want you to have a fast-metabolism smoothie and a muscle-building smoothie.

Muscle-Building Shake

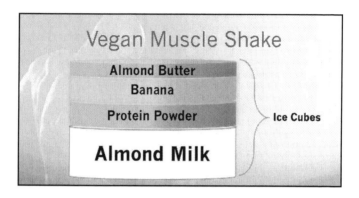

Here's a simple template or recipe that works well. Since ideally you'll need extra protein, extra carbohydrates, and extra fat, this is a combination I love that is delicious and will help you build a lot of muscle quickly:

1. In a blender, add one to two scoops of your favorite plant-based protein powder.

2. Add some almond milk.

3. Add a scoop of natural peanut butter or almond butter.

4. Add a couple of bananas.

5. Add ice.

6. Blend for two minutes.

Now you've got a delicious protein shake that tastes like a milkshake. Drink it, along with a fast-metabolism smoothie, and you have a perfect combination for building muscle.

If you feel like chewing, and having a meal on a plate instead of a smoothie, you can take the same approach when choosing muscle-building ingredients to build a meal.

Start with a basic fast-metabolism meal:

1. Add a serving of beans, rice, or lentils.

2. Add whole, sprouted, organic bread, like Ezekiel bread (or even make a sandwich).

3. Add good fats, such as avocado, natural peanut butter, or almond butter.

The choices are vast. Try different combinations and find out which ones you like. Most people love eating muscle-building meals because they're able to eat foods that they normally wouldn't eat when they're trying to lose fat. The good news is, this is going to help your body look and feel even better and stronger, and make your muscles even bigger.

Creating a Muscle-Building Meal

Step 1. Eat a fast-metabolism meal or smoothie until satisfied.

Step 2. Eat a high-carbohydrate food until full.

Step 3. Eat a high-protein food until uncomfortably full.

Yes, you are eating all of this as a single meal!

Sample Muscle-Building Meals

Fast-metabolism smoothie until satisfied + Ezekiel bread and almond butter sandwich until full + tofu until uncomfortably full

Or

Fast-metabolism meal until satisfied + brown rice until full + vegan protein powder until uncomfortably full

Or

Fast-metabolism smoothie until satisfied + vegan muscle shake until uncomfortably full (vegan muscle shake contains both carbs and high protein)

Or

Fast-metabolism meal until satisfied + fruit platter until full + tempeh until uncomfortably full

Creating Your Muscle-Building Meal Plan

Creating your muscle-building meal plan is similar to creating your fat-loss meal plan, except you're just adding more ingredients. Start by creating a base of your fast-metabolism meals and smoothies. Then make multiple servings at one time of your favorite complex or muscle-building carbohydrates. For example, instead of making one serving of rice, make six or seven servings at one time, so you have enough for several days. If you're making one serving of beans, make eight to ten servings at once so you have plenty of good, complex, muscle-building carbohydrates to go.

When it comes to protein, do the same thing. Make several servings of protein instead of one. If you're cutting up or baking tofu, make four to eight servings and store them in the refrigerator so you can grab them and go if needed.

And when it comes to creating smoothies, there's no reason you couldn't make several batches of muscle-building smoothies to go.

What's better than one muscle-building smoothie?

Five or six! Put them in jars and store them in the refrigerator, and they'll last for at least a day or two, depending on how cool the refrigerator is.

My suggestion is to always buy in bulk and prepare in bulk. It's a great time-saver and ensures you have your meals whenever you need them.

One of the biggest pitfalls when it comes to building muscle is nutrition. The most common reason most people are not able to build muscle quickly or as much as they want is because they're simply not eating enough. The problem people have with muscle-building nutrition is the opposite of the problem they have when trying to lose weight or lose fat. When it comes to losing fat, the biggest mistake people make is they eat too much. When it comes to building muscle, the biggest mistake people make is they eat too little.

It's not easy to build muscle, because you must eat to an uncomfortable fullness every single meal. You can never let yourself go hungry; in fact, you should force yourself to eat even when you're not hungry. That's not easy, and it can take a toll on your mental capacity after time. So you have to stay strong, and you have to be willing to feel uncomfortable in order to grow, and that means feeling fuller after eating than you've ever felt in your entire life. If you go through a week of muscle-building nutrition and you feel like you can't look at or think of food, you're doing it right.

That's when you want to pat yourself on the back and say, "Good job, I'm growing—literally."

MUSCLE-BUILDING EXERCISE

The second component necessary to build muscle is muscle-building exercise. You must combine that with muscle-building nutrition for muscle to grow. One of the biggest mistakes people make is they do muscle-building exercise, but they don't have the correct nutrition to build the muscle. Muscle-building exercise sets the body up to be able to build muscle, but it's the nutrition that actually puts the muscle on.

Conversely, if you eat for muscle gain, but you don't work out for muscle gain, your body will get bigger, but as a result of body fat, and that's not what you want. When building muscle, you want to get bigger from muscle and not fat. That's where the muscle-building exercises make a difference in how well, how much, and how quickly you will build muscle.

Characteristics of Muscle-Building Exercise

The intent, when performing muscle-building exercises, is to create as much damage as possible across all the muscle tissue that you are exercising. It's the damage that releases the hormones that signal your body to begin the muscle-rebuilding process. When you provide your body with an excess of raw materials and nutrients to build the muscle, you will get an excess of muscle when your body rebuilds it. To do that, you are going to focus all your energy on a narrow group of muscles.

When you are trying to lose fat, you're training every single muscle in the body at once. When you exercise for building muscle, you're concentrating all your mental and physical energy on one or two different muscles or muscle groups at once, and that's it. This allows for more damage to occur, which is what you want.

You're going to use workout strategies like pyramids and drop-sets, and that's going to allow you to work the entire muscle.

Your muscles contain different muscle fibers, and those muscle fibers come in different categories and different types:

- Some muscle fiber types only get damaged with high repetitions and lighter weights.

- Some muscle fiber types only get damaged with fewer repetitions and heavier weights.

- Some muscle fiber types only get damaged with medium repetitions and medium weights.

This means that you need to use a variety of different weights and reps, always going to muscular failure to create the damage across the *entire* muscle, not just one part of it. One mistake people make in trying to use exercise to build muscle is they only stick within a narrow rep range. Typically, they do eight to twelve repetitions, which is a moderate amount of repetitions, and only damages a moderate amount of the muscle. If you want to build muscle the fastest way possible, you want to work the entire muscle. We're going to be using pyramids and drop-sets to achieve that efficiently and quickly.

Pyramids

An example of a pyramid chest workout would involve using a bench press and starting with the highest weight that forces you to quit between twenty and thirty reps. If you don't have a spotter, use a smith machine.

Increase the weight by twenty pounds every consecutive set, banging out as many reps as you possibly can. Keep doing this until you get to a weight that forces you to quit after two or three reps. Then, take off twenty pounds after each consecutive set and continue to bang out as many reps as possible until you come back to your starting weight.

That is a complete pyramid and will thoroughly train all the muscle fiber types in your chest.

Drop Sets

An example of a drop set for the biceps would be using the heaviest weight possible for two to five repetitions of a biceps cable curl. Then, after reaching muscular failure, immediately decrease the weight by one to two plates and bang out as many reps as you can.

Once you reach muscular failure, immediately decrease the weight and repeat.

How many sets you do depends on how much pain you are willing to take. My drop sets typically go for about five sets. I will go until I've reach a total of twenty to thirty repetitions, so I know that I've trained all of my muscle fiber types.

Muscle-Building Exercises

The four most important exercises for building muscle are:

- Deadlifts and all variations
- Squats and all variations
- Any form of press
- Any form of row

A common misconception about bodybuilding is that you should do ten to fifteen different exercises whenever you work out. The truth is, you don't. You only need these four; that's it. These four will exercise all the different muscles in your body in the most effective way possible. You will get far greater results concentrating all your efforts on just these four simple exercises than you would if you did fifteen or twenty-five exercises for all the different body parts.

Exercise 1: Deadlift

A deadlift is an exercise where you simply pick up a weight from the floor and bring it to your hips. Then you set it back down and repeat.

Variations of deadlifts include:

- Barbell deadlifts
- Dumbbell deadlifts
- Machine deadlifts
- Romanian deadlifts
- Keystone deadlifts

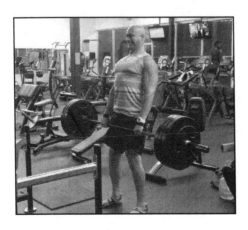

Exercise 2: Squat

A squat is done by lowering your body with your legs positioned as if you were going to sit. How far you go down will depend on your skill level and the condition of your joints. Most people perform squats by going down until their thighs are parallel.

Variations of the squat include:

- Barbell squats
- Front squats
- Machine hack squats
- Machine leg press

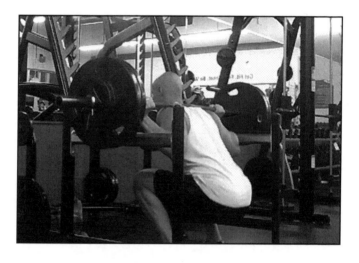

Exercise 3: Press

Pressing exercises are done with the upper body, in which you push the weight or resistance in any direction away from your body. These exercises can be done with barbells, dumbbells, or machines.

They include:

- Bench presses
- Incline presses
- Decline presses
- Military presses

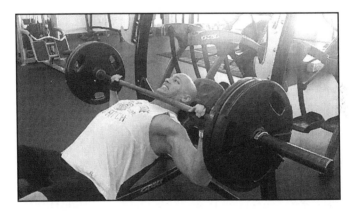

Exercise 4: Row

Rows are a form of exercise done with the upper body, in which you pull the weight or resistance in any direction toward your body. These exercises include:

- Barbell bent rows
- Dumbbell rows
- Pull-ups
- Pull-downs
- Machine rows
- High cable rows
- Upright rows

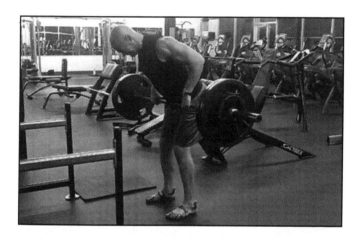

Creating Your Muscle-Building Workout Routine

When I was studying to be a personal trainer, there was a section in every single one of my personal training texts on building muscle that suggested a certain number of days per week to concentrate on building muscle, how often you should work each muscle part, how many sets, and so on. I noticed, as I achieved one certification after another, that the guidelines were all similar. But what was interesting was that the results I was getting with my clients were *not* similar, even though I was putting the same guidelines to work.

I discovered that prescribing a number of reps, sets, and frequency just does not work with everybody, because our genetics and recovery abilities are different. And everyone's ability and speed to heal is different for many reasons, including:

- Genetics
- Stress level
- Sleeping habits
- Nutrition quality

So, the best way to plan your workouts is to set up your four exercises, go into the gym on day one, do the first exercise, and pyramid them. Do as many of them as you possibly can. Just commit to doing the first and second exercises. Do as many of those as you possibly can, until you can't do any more. When you get to the point where you can't do any more, if you have any energy left, do the third exercise. And if you can't do it, that's okay:

- Go home.
- Get some rest.
- Go back the next day.
- Pick up where you left off.

The real key to designing your workouts is to perform each of the four exercises, or movements, as soon as you can. You might find that you'll be able to do crunches every day, to full failure, but you'll only be able to do drop-sets and pyramid push-and-pull movements every other day. That's perfect, because it means you're working optimally to your body's recovery ability.

You might find you can only do squatting movements and deadlifts once every seven to ten days. And that's perfect, too, because it's based 100 percent on how quickly those muscles are able to fully recover. That's the secret when designing your routine: let your body tell you when it's ready to do each of the four exercises.

Document everything you are doing in the gym — write down every set, every rep, and every exercise you do. You'll be able to track what you're doing. When you combine the correct muscle-building exercises with the right nutrition, you should notice that every time you come back, you can do more, either in terms of repetition or a certain amount of weight. You want to see that you're getting stronger every single time. That's why it's so important to document. So again, you're not going to walk in with a prescribed number of sets and reps, but you are going to write down what you do, so you can see your progress.

Are you increasing the reps and weights from workout to workout?

When measuring your results while building muscle, you want to use the scale. It will be your best friend. Your weight should be going up, week after week, if you're really building muscle and putting on mass. That's the consequence of adding tissue. You're going to add a little bit of fat, but you will also add a lot of muscle.

You will also notice your strength and endurance increasing. If they're not, that usually means you're not eating enough. Another thing you want to do to make sure you are achieving progress is to take before-and-after pictures. I recommend that you take a new picture of your body and compare it against the previous picture every two weeks. When building muscles, two weeks is a good period in which to see the difference in body transformation. Taking pictures one week apart might not be enough time to see a noticeable change. I also recommend flexing in the photos; when your muscles are flexed, it's much easier to see how much they've grown.

PUTTING IT INTO PRACTICE

Now that you understand how to eat and work out to build muscle, let's talk about how to set yourself up for success, so you can build all the muscle you want.

Muscle-Building Tools

The first step in building muscle is having the proper workout tools. You should decide if you're going to perform the muscle-building exercises at home or at a gym. I highly recommend you get a gym membership, because you'll have access to trainers and spotters who can help you. Doing pyramids isn't easy, and it's also going to be hard at times. Also, you want to make sure that you're 100 percent safe. I recommend that you always use a spotter whenever doing free weights exercises in which the weight or bar is positioned over your body. Since you'll be working to absolute muscular failure most of the time, you may not have the strength to push the bar or weight away from your body. I've seen people get stuck under the bench press machine. It's not pretty. Plus, with a gym membership you have access to equipment that you typically wouldn't have room for in your home.

But if you're not going to join a gym, make sure you get the right equipment, including:

- Dumbbells
- An adjustable bench
- Weight plates and bar
- Protective rubber floor mats
- Gloves
- Lifting strap
- Lifting belt

Dumbbells

I recommend you get a set of PowerBlock dumbbells. These are adjustable dumbbells that allow you to set the weight anywhere between two-and-a-half pounds to 125 pounds, and they take up very little space. A set typically runs about $750.00.

Adjustable Bench

I also recommend you get an adjustable bench. You can find them at any sporting goods store, or the sporting goods sections of Wal-Mart and Target, for about $100.00 to $200.00. To perform deadlifts and squats, you'll need an Olympic bar with a squatting cage. Residential versions take up less space than the big ones you see at the gym, and they're very affordable.

Weight Plates and Bar, and Protective Mats

And let's not forget the weight plates. Make sure that you have the proper tools and equipment to be able to perform the lifts. You can find Olympic weight and bar combo-sets that contain about 300 pounds of weight for around $300.00. You're going to need space to set it up, so use either a room in your house, or many folks like to use their garages as their personal gyms. Avoid using an upstairs room, unless you get protective mats. If a few hundred pounds come crashing down, it can damage the floor. Thick rubber mats will protect your floors. When I owned a fitness studio, we covered the entire floor of our facility with ¾ inch rubber mats designed for weightlifting. They come in 4 x 6 foot sections and cost around $100.00 per mat.

Gloves and Lifting Straps

Other great tools to have are gloves and lifting straps. Sometimes, your forearms will give out faster than your back and leg muscles. You don't want that to stop you. I highly recommend you perform forearm-strengthening exercises. Often your back and legs can grow stronger than your forearms can handle. Using lifting straps and gloves can increase your grip and comfort, and help you lift the bar when your forearms are giving out. That allows you to exercise your muscles to full exhaustion, even after your forearm muscles are ready to give out.

Lifting Belt

Lastly, don't forget a lifting belt. It's always good to have a lifting belt, just in case. Again, your legs and back muscles will get strong fast, usually outpacing the speed that the smaller muscles that support your spine and joints gain strength. A lifting belt can add an additional layer of support and stability to your lower spine, allowing you to lift more weight safely.

You don't want to be dependent on the lifting belt, but you do want to have it available whenever you are lifting your heaviest weight for the first time, and you haven't allowed the time to be able to develop the proper strength through your back and core. The lifting belt will be able to protect your spine and lower back muscles from injury. Staying injury-free is key to building and keeping strong muscles over the long term.

Scheduling: Making the Time and Making It Happen

When it comes to building muscle, consistency is absolutely key. Unfortunately, you can't go to the gym and in one workout build all the muscle you want and keep it forever. If you don't continue to work out and perform muscle-building exercises, your muscles will adapt by getting smaller. Your muscles will be only as strong as you are forcing them to be. You don't want that to happen, so make sure you allocate time in your day and schedule to perform a proper muscle-building workout.

You want to allocate anywhere between forty-five and ninety minutes per workout. I would say seventy-five minutes, on average, to be safe. That's plenty of time for you to perform the pyramids and drop-sets, and gives you plenty of rest in between. You are going to be performing a large number of sets, especially as you get in better shape. You will move through your workout more quickly as your cardiovascular endurance increases, but you still want to make sure you give yourself a proper amount of time. This is when having your own home setup can be handy, because it requires no additional time for getting to the gym and back. When the gym is right there in your own home, it's just steps away.

If you've ever heard that it's important to have a meal before your workout and immediately after, I've got good news for you. It's absolutely *not* necessary at all. You can perform a muscle-building workout on an empty stomach and still build all the muscle you want, as quickly as you want to. Not only have I tested *not* eating a pre- or post-workout meal, I have plenty of friends who don't and continue to win bodybuilding competitions all over the world. So, don't let that stop you. Schedule your workout time when it's most convenient for you. Just make sure that you do it consistently, and you have it scheduled in your calendar so nothing can get in the way.

When your muscles hurt so badly that you feel you can't even get up to work out, that's a good time to take a rest day. Take rest days as often as you need to, but not when you *feel* like it. Take them when your muscles *need* to. When your muscles are telling you it's time to rest, then rest. It's okay. You may average about four to five workouts per week, and that's perfect. I only worked out an average of four days per week and gained 10.1 pounds in just twenty-eight days, nearly doubling in strength during that time. I did zero planning for pre- or post-workout meals. If I ate, it was when I felt like it.

Measuring Your Results

When measuring your muscle-building results, you will need:

- Body weight scale
- Tape measure
- Camera
- Log book

Body Weight Scale

When building muscle, the scale is an incredibly valuable tool. Building muscle is a process of adding more tissue than you currently have. You want to see your body weight going up as a result of increased muscle tissue from muscle-building workouts and muscle-building nutrition. If you're eating to uncomfortable fullness and performing muscle-building exercises to complete muscular failure, you will see your weight go up in a good way.

Step on the scale every morning after you go to the bathroom, before you have had anything to eat or drink. Record your body weight along with the date. Do this every day and you should notice your body weight measurements fluctuating up and down. If your lowest weight each week is higher than the previous week, and if your highest weight each week is higher than the previous week, then you are doing it right. If you are not seeing your highest highs and lowest lows getting heavier each week, the remedy is simple. Eat more until your weight increases every week.

Tape Measure

Bigger muscles will also mean bigger measurements. If you increase the size of the muscles in your arms, your arms will measure bigger. If you increase the size of the muscles in your legs, your legs will measure bigger, too. Using a tape measure is a great way to see progress in building muscle on a body-part-by-body-part basis.

The best places to measure muscle growth are your arms, shoulders, legs, and chest.

Arms

Flex your right arm by making a big muscle. Then wrap the measuring tape all the way around your bicep and tricep and measure the widest area as you flex your bicep. Repeat for the other arm.

Shoulders

Have a partner help you wrap the measuring tape around your whole body, starting from the widest point of one shoulder, around the widest point of your other shoulder, and back again. The measuring tape will go across your back and your chest. Make sure the tape is steady and parallel to the floor and record the measurement.

Legs

Make a muscle with your leg by straightening it as much as you can. Wrap the measuring tape around the widest part, making it go around your hamstring and back to the front of your quadriceps. Make sure the measuring tape is level and parallel to the ground and record the measurement. Repeat for the other leg.

Perform these measurements every two to four weeks. If your measurements are increasing, you're doing everything right.

If a measurement is not increasing, but your bodyweight is, then you need to perform more sets on those muscles. Increase your sets and work those muscles more frequently.

If a measurement is not increasing and your bodyweight is not either, then you need to eat more and possibly exercise those body parts more.

Camera

Using pictures and video are powerful ways to see your progress. Make sure you are in a well-lit area. Position your camera so you can see your whole body from head to toe. Wear a bathing suit or workout gear that clearly reveals most of your body. Take pictures from the front, sides, and back. When using video, simply press record and slowly turn 360 degrees in place. Take and compare pictures and video every four weeks.

Strength Logs

Recording every rep, set, and weight during each workout is one of the most effective ways to measure progress when you are building muscle. From week to week, it is difficult to see how much your muscles are growing. They need to grow several pounds larger before their progress is visibly noticeable. However, you can observe your muscle growth by seeing their strength and endurance. Muscles that become bigger *have* to be stronger and have better endurance.

By keeping track of how much weight you used for each set of each exercise and how many reps you completed to muscular failure, you can begin observing your muscular gains in the form of strength and endurance increases.

Muscular growth is occurring if you are regularly exceeding how much weight you are able to lift for a given number of repetitions. This means you are getting stronger. Growth is also occurring if you are able to exceed your greatest number of reps at a given weight.

To log your workouts, write down the name of the exercise followed by the number of reps and weight that you accomplished: exercise reps at [x] weight.

Try to do this following each set. Here's what a sample log might look like:

VEGAN MUSCLE SYSTEM

DAY 18   DATE 12/18/2014

Exercise name/variation	SQUAT	PRESS	ROW	DEADLIFT
	LB press	OH shoulder press	Lat pulldown	
SET 1	20×180	25×35 lb	14×120 lb	
SET 2	18×225	14×40 lb	12×140 lb	
SET 3	15×270	10×45 lb	9×160 lb	
SET 4	10×315	7×50 lb	15×135	
SET 5	9×360	5×55 lb	...	
SET 6	7×405	4×60 AU	...	
SET 7	4×450	3×65 AU		
SET 8	3×500	4×65		
SET 9	2×500	3×65		
SET 10	3×450	3×60		
SET 11	4×405	5×55		
SET 12	4×360	3×55		
SET 13	6×315	4×50		
SET 14	5×270	5×45		
SET 15	6×225	6×40		
SET 16	9×180	7×35		
SET 17				

I write the letters PR — personal record — next to a set that exceeds my previous best. Again, I'm counting a personal record as every time I'm able to exceed my highest weight for a given number of reps or when I'm able to exceed my highest number of reps for a given weight.

If you are eating enough to build muscle and using the workout guidelines I've laid out for you in this chapter, you should be setting PRs at virtually every single workout.

Case Studies

These are the results I achieved after just twenty-eight days:

> Weight: +10.1lbs
> Waist: -1"
> Biceps: +1.25" each
> Body fat: -1 percent

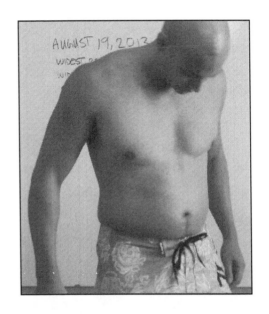

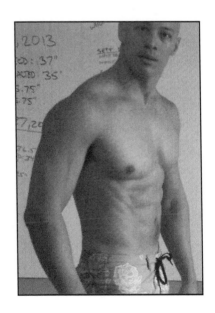

The muscle and strength was coming on fast, and it was so easy and simple to keep going, so I did. I kept this up for several more weeks. The results were greater than I've ever achieved in my life.

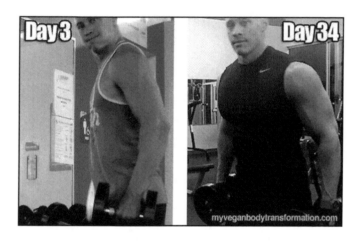

Six Weeks Later

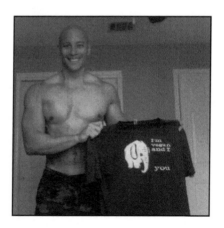

Allen Bulked Up and Shrunk His Waist

Weight: +2.2 lbs
Body Fat: -1.0 percent
Chest: +1.13"
Left Arm: +0.25"
Right Arm: +1.0"
Hips/Butt: +0.25"
Waist: -2.13"
Left Thigh: +2.25"
Right Thigh: +2.0"
Left Calf: -0.5"
Right Calf: -0.38"
Shoulders: +0.38"

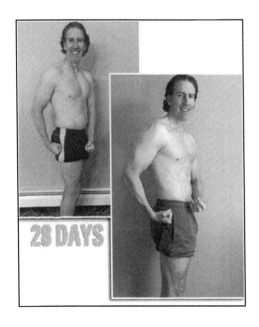

Joe Gained Nineteen Pounds and Dropped Body Fat!

Weight: +19.0 lbs

Body Fat: -2.2 %

Left Arm: +1.25"

Right Arm: +1.0"

Hips/Butt: +1.0"

Waist: -0.5"

Left Thigh: +0.75"

Right Thigh: +0.75"

Shoulders: +2.0"

"I did not expect to gain nineteen pounds and two-and-a-half inches on my chest and shoulders! I'm looking a lot buffer than I was a month ago and all my friends have been absolutely astounded at the amount of muscle I've been able to achieve. I am more energized and physically motivated than I can remember being in years. I can't possible stress the effectiveness and awesomeness of this program enough! Thanks so much; I couldn't be more grateful!"

-Joe Nash

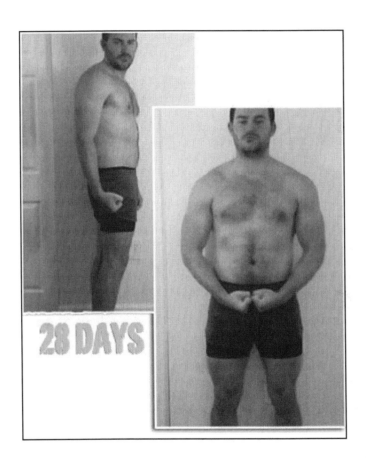

Jen Added Caps to Her Shoulders!

Body Fat: -2.0 percent
Left Arm: +0.25"
Right Arm: +0.25"
Hips/Butt: +1.5"
Waist: +0.25"
Left Thigh: +0.25"
Right Thigh: +0.25"
Shoulders: +0.75"

It's pretty incredible. This program shatters the misconceptions of muscle building on a vegan diet. I am extremely happy about my results. Within the first two weeks, people in my office were noticing my arms through my shirt. I have definitely built muscle and feel so strong; normally at this weight I would feel very heavy and slow! This program has given me a renewed fire to push myself to my limits. I had just done personal training sessions once a week and that is just not enough to build the kind of muscle I did on this program. I definitely would recommend this program, especially to those who are not vegan already.

- Jen Salik

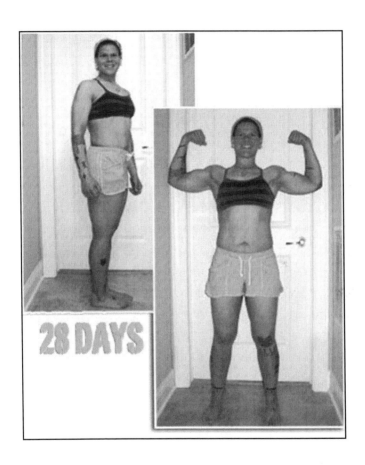

Final Thoughts about Putting It Into Practice

One of my favorite aspects of building muscle on a vegan diet, the way that I just showed you, is it will raise your metabolism. So many people are amazed when they see me working out at the gym, and they see how strong I am. But when they find out that I am 100 percent vegan and eating only a half to a third of the protein that most people my size eat, and still creating gains twice as fast as them, they are blown away. Be prepared to get a lot of compliments. Also, be prepared to be accused of using steroids, because the results come very quickly, faster than what most people are used to seeing. Just be prepared to smile and share this information with anybody who's curious, especially the naysayers. You'll be surprised how many people will be influenced in a positive way. I've had many people go vegan just from watching my rapid gains in the gym and talking to me. Take lots of pictures, post them on Facebook, and be an inspiration to the world. This is how you create change!

CHAPTER *FIVE*

Having It All and Keeping It Forever

THE INCONVENIENT TRUTHS ABOUT FAT LOSS AND MUSCLE BUILDING

First, congratulations for making it this far. If you've read all the chapters up to here, go ahead and give yourself a pat on the back, because not a lot of people make it this far. Body transformation is an educational process at first. Then, it's a doing process. If you've taken the time to read everything in this book, you now are familiar with what it takes to build muscle and lose fat.

Now let's put it all together. But first, I want to tell you why you don't want to focus on fat loss or muscle building alone for a long period of time. There are some unwanted consequences connected to those two things, which I want to help you understand and avoid.

The Effects on the Thyroid From Prolonged Fat Loss

To lose fat quickly, you'll be performing fat-loss exercise workouts as well as eating a fast-metabolism diet, which is going to put you on a lower-than-normal caloric intake. And you're going to be burning more calories than you normally would if you weren't exercising like this, so it's going to put you at a caloric deficit overall. Over time, with a caloric deficit caused by eating less or exercising more, your thyroid function begins to decrease. When that happens, unfortunately it slows your metabolism, which is *not* what you want. You want to lose fat consistently and easily without any slowing of your results.

You may have noticed that people often get great results in the beginning of their weight-loss programs, and then the results start to taper off. Maybe that's happened to you. Many folks believe that they don't lose weight as easily as they used to because of their age or their genetics. I'm here to tell you that's not true! It's just simply that your body is good at adapting to what you feed it and what you consistently force it to do. Even if you're eating plenty of nourishing foods while exercising, your fat loss will eventually slow down, as your body tries to function close to the way it was. It wants to maintain a certain equilibrium.

Your body doesn't make drastic changes for the long-term. It wants to adapt to a changing environment, and then keep itself the same. If you're feeding yourself a highly nourishing diet and exercising regularly, but you're not losing weight as fast as you used to, it doesn't mean that your body's not doing what it's supposed to. It means it's *really* good at doing what it's supposed to. Over time, your body finds creative ways to get away with creating as little change as possible, because change takes energy. Your body is always looking for the path of least resistance. If you train and eat for fat loss over a long period of time, you will eventually notice your fat loss slow down. This happens even if you still have many more pounds to lose.

If there's one primary organ that controls your body's overall metabolism, it's your thyroid. When your thyroid is functioning normally, it's very easy for you to lose body fat. When there's a problem with the thyroid, it is usually under-functioning. This tends to make weight loss very slow, often with the inconvenient effect of the body gaining weight more easily with less food.

Let's discuss the inconvenient truth around muscle building, and then we'll dive into what to do about the slowdown that happens when trying to lose fat over a long period of time.

The Effects on Body Fat From Prolonged Muscle Gain

The inconvenient truth about building muscle is that you can't build muscle fast without adding some body fat. That's because the hormones involved with the creation of more muscle tissue are also the same hormones that are present when body fat is created. One of those primary hormones is insulin. Insulin is what helps you build muscle in a big way; it is an amazing muscle-building hormone, and without it you can't build much muscle at all.

Unfortunately, it's also the hormone that stimulates the growth and creation of fat. To build muscle, you know you must do muscle-building exercises, but when you go on a high-calorie diet, which you have to, it's impossible to calculate the exact amount of excess food needed to be able to build just muscle without any fat. In fact, it's not even possible. Even if you had the right amount of food calculated, some of it will always go to the creation of fat and the creation of muscle as long as you're doing muscle-building exercises. The key is trying to minimize the amount of fat you create while trying to maximize the amount of muscle, knowing that creating fat is unavoidable when you are building muscle. But that's okay; I'm going to show you how to get around these things.

Introduction to Zig-Zag Dieting

A long time ago, I was awarded my first fitness training certification by the International Sports Sciences Association, which was founded by Dr. Fred Hatfield, one of the greatest fitness training icons in the fitness industry. He is regarded among professionals as one of the smartest, most revolutionary body transformation experts in the world. He created something called the zig-zag eating and training strategy; he called it the zig-zag diet. It's about being able to separate your fat-loss days and your muscle-building days, on separate days of the week.

On certain days, you concentrate on losing fat, and other days on building muscle. The idea on fat-loss days is to maximize fat loss and minimize muscle loss. On the muscle-building days—the *up-zag* days—you concentrate on building muscle and maximizing the amount of muscle gain while minimizing the fat gain. So, at the end of the week, the result would be a net gain in muscle, and a net loss in body fat. That's the strategy you are going to use to create the body you want, whether it be gaining weight in muscle without gaining the fat, losing weight without losing any muscle, or just maintaining so that you can continue to get leaner and stronger.

CREATING YOUR DREAM BODY BLUEPRINT

I hope you're excited, because you are *so* close to creating your entire plan! The plan shows how you can lose all the weight you want, coming 100 percent from fat, while preserving the muscle that you have, or maintaining your current weight while reducing fat and building the same amount of muscle. Whichever you want to do, I'll show you how to create the blueprint to make it happen.

Zig-Zag Plan for Weight Maintenance

Weight maintenance is one of the best places for anyone to start if you've never done a zig-zag plan before. The goal is to build muscle and lose an equal amount of fat. An example is to gain five pounds of muscle and lose five pounds of fat. If you do that, your weight will stay exactly the same, although your body fat percentage will be significantly lower, meaning that you would look stronger, leaner, and fitter. You'll look like you weigh less, although you will remain the same.

To achieve this, perform an equal number of *up* days and an equal number of *down* days over the course of a week. An up day is a muscle-building day, so on those days you do only muscle-building exercises and eat using the muscle-building nutrition strategy. Down days are those days when you're only going to do fat-loss exercises and eat according to the fat-loss nutrition strategy. You should notice on the scale that on up days your weight goes up, and on down days your weight goes down. At the end of the week, there's virtually no change in your body weight, although there will be a big difference in how much more muscular and leaner you look.

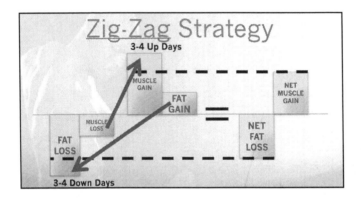

When you are structuring your up and down days, all that matters is having an equal number of up and down days. Just zig-zag; up and down and up and down and up and down. Or, if it's more convenient, Monday through Wednesday can be up days, and Thursday through Saturday down days. Then just repeat the sequence from Sunday: three ups, three downs. Choose whatever order works the best for you, as long as you are averaging an equal number of up and down days. You can even do up weeks and down weeks, whatever your personal preference.

Zig-Zag Plan for Fat Loss

The zig-zag plan for fat loss is the fastest method of losing body weight from fat because you combine up days with mostly down days to maintain thyroid function and keep your metabolism high to maximize the rate of fat loss. The goal for the fat-loss zig-zag plan is to lose the greatest amount of weight from fat and build back any muscle you might have lost along the way. For example, if you lose seven pounds over a few weeks, but two of them are from muscle, the goal would be to build those extra two pounds of muscle back, so that by the end of every week, you end up with a net loss in body fat, and no change in muscle.

These plans are typically five to six down days, with one or two up days. If you follow that plan, what's most convenient for people is making Sunday through Thursday the down days, and Friday and Saturday as the up days.

Why?

I love going out to eat on Fridays and Saturdays, and since my Fridays and Saturdays are up days, I can choose to eat whatever I want—on top of having my smoothies and making sure I get my protein—because you can build a lot of muscle when you have an excess amount of food. Those are perfect days to go out to eat. You also won't feel like you're depriving and starving yourself week after week, because long-term dieting and restriction can burn you out emotionally. This is a way to minimize the burnout while keeping your metabolism high and losing a huge amount of fat.

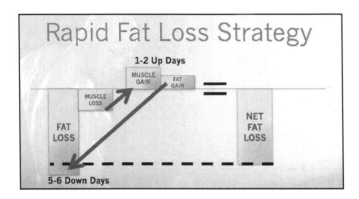

Zig-Zag Plan for Muscle Gain

The other zig-zag strategy is gaining weight from muscle. The goal for this strategy is to create a net gain in muscle with absolutely no change in body fat by the end of the week. You want to build muscle without putting on any fat. This will, again, lower your body fat percentage while increasing your weight. This is great for anybody who wants to gain weight the healthy way.

The typical strategy for this zig-zag plan is five to six up days, combined with one or two down days. You'll spend five or six days building as much muscle as you possibly can, knowing that you're going to add a little bit of body fat. Now, if you follow the strategies that we taught you in the muscle-building section, with your green smoothies and good carbohydrates, and doing nothing but muscle-building exercise (and a lot of it), you will maximize your muscle building while minimizing your fat gain. Then, you'll add one or two down days of fat-loss exercise and fat-loss nutrition, which will remove any excess fat you gained during that cycle, leaving you with more muscle and the same amount of fat. This will decrease your body fat percentage while increasing your weight.

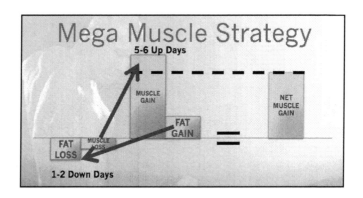

Results

Here are my results after just seven days. I'm not kidding—just seven days of applying the strategy of three to four up days and three to four down days. I basically alternated between up and down days and this is what happened after just one week.

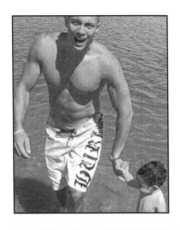
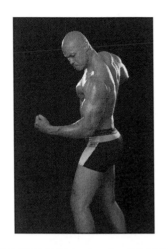

Before	Seven Days Later

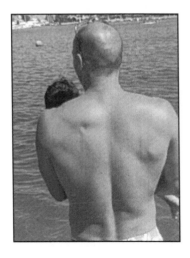
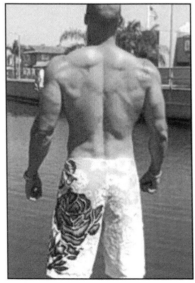

Before	Seven Days Later

Creating Your Zig-Zag

Now it's time to create *your* zig-zag plan. Step one is deciding on the goal you would like to achieve.

Would you like to weigh exactly the same but replace your fat with muscle?

If that's the case, choose the maintenance zig-zag plan: an equal number of up and down days. That would be three to four down days, and three to four up days every single week.

Or is your goal to lose weight?

If that's the goal, choose the fast fat-loss zig-zag strategy. That's five to six down days, and one to two up days.

Or is your goal to gain weight?

If that's the case, choose one to two down days and five to six up days.

Use the sample Monday-through-Sunday schedule below, and schedule your up and down days over the course of the week.

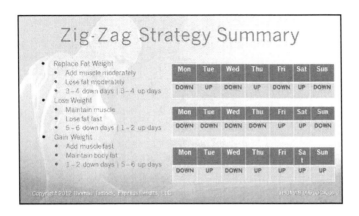

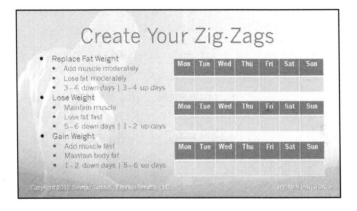

Now you know how to build muscle, how to lose fat, the nutrition and workout strategies for both, and you have created your blueprint. All that's left is for you to put it into action. Use the blueprint above as your daily guide for success. Make sure you follow our advice for scheduling and making it happen, measure your results on a regular basis, and watch the miracles occur! Please feel free to post your updates online by going to SmoothieShred.com. We'd love to see them, and we'd love to cheer you on.

METABOLIC NINJA TACTICS

For many years, I've had clients share with me their frustration around maintaining eating and exercise routines during certain events in their lives, like parties and holidays. These sometimes stressed out my clients, because they wanted to be able to celebrate and enjoy the food typically served at those events, but they didn't want to screw up the results of their diet. Well, I have good news for you. You've learned enough now to understand how your body and metabolism work. You can enjoy these events and still look and feel better afterward. Let's dive in to some amazing ninja tactics you can use to get your metabolism to work for you and not against you.

Holiday Parties

Holidays and holiday parties happen in the course of everyone's life — when there's a plethora of food and drink that wouldn't be on any sort of rapid fat-loss or muscle-building plan. But that's okay. All you need to do to end those days better than when you started them is to use an up day. On those occasions, make sure you do a muscle-building workout and consume fast-metabolism smoothies as your foundation, consume your protein and fats, and then give yourself permission to eat whatever else you want. All that excess food and nutrients — even if it's candy, dessert, or not-so-healthy food — will go toward your muscle-building efforts. You will gain some fat, but that's exactly why you have a blueprint; your down days will take care of that. Adding more nutrients to your body will help you build more muscle as long as you perform a muscle-building workout on those days.

Again, don't stress about holiday parties. You can have your cake *and* build some muscle, too. Make it an up day, and you'll never feel guilty about enjoying yourself.

Falling Off the Wagon

What often can happen is people fall off the wagon. That's right, they go completely off the nutrition plan, the workout plan, or both. This might last for several days, or possibly several weeks. It can have a large emotional effect and a big effect on the body. Many emotions are connected to exercise and body image. The normal response is to feel guilty. However, my advice is don't feel guilty; allow those feelings to come and go.

Just sit back and observe, and ask yourself a question: "Is this supporting me or not supporting me right now?"

That's it; it's not whether it's good or bad, but just whether it's supporting you or not.

When you're ready to come back, I recommend one of two strategies, and you can choose the one that feels best. One, you can go into the fat-replacement strategy, easing into it by doing up and down days. If you have a tendency to fall off the wagon by overeating, that's fine. If you use a fat-replacement strategy, then you'll be giving yourself plenty of up days to nourish your body and get yourself back in a state where you don't feel deprived, but you start seeing results right away.

The second strategy, if you have a tendency of not working out, is to use the fat-loss strategy, which is five to six down days, and only one or two up days a week. This will help you get very lean and defined right away, and fitting better in your clothes is an instant confidence booster. I recommend you do whichever plan feels right to you.

Getting Sick

Almost like clockwork, every year nearly everyone I know gets hit with the flu or a cold that takes them out of the game. You miss the gym for several days, and especially if you get the flu, it takes you out of your eating strategy for several days. The last time I had the flu, which was a long time ago, I didn't feel like eating for at least four or five days. I had just some basic vegetable broth and that was it.

In a case like that, in which it wasn't easy for me to do an up day, I would start with a fat-replacement strategy, to let my stomach ease into eating regular food. I would do three to five down days in a row, and then introduce an up day, going easy of course. The low frequency of up days allowed my stomach and my body to ease into it while also getting in shape. The fast-metabolism smoothies are the perfect cure to get back into shape after being sick.

If you go through several days when you can't eat, and you have a strong stomach and you don't mind eating a lot of food when the sickness is over, then go right into the mega-muscle strategy. This means doing five or six up days followed by one or two down days. If you're able to stomach food, that will go a long way to replenishing all the nutrients and muscle glycogen that you lost while you were sick. This will help you get your strength and muscle back in no time.

You now have all the tools you need to be able to succeed. You know what to do in just about any scenario or situation. Now is the time for you to make it happen.

Conclusion

Congratulations, you've made it! You've read the entire book and you know what it will take to transform your body. You know how to:

- Raise your metabolism
- Lose all the body fat you want
- Build all the muscle that you want
- Maintain it forever

Now, it's your turn to make it happen. We've gone over all the strategies and tactics to integrate it into your life, and it's time for you to put it into action and get the results. I am so excited to see what your results will be.

I'll tell you right now, it's not going to be easy. But, using the tools I've given you, it will be easier than anything you've done before to get these results. The results are going to be amazing, if you stay committed to it. They will absolutely blow your mind!

This is not just about looking better, and getting stronger and leaner. It is about living a long, happy, and healthy life. It's about increasing your energy, and it's also about sharing this information and being a role model for other people.

Have you had the experience of watching someone in your life make a change and see them achieve great results?

It's inspirational, and that's the impact you're going to have on others. It's so important that you do this not only for yourself, but for others around you, too. You can serve to be an inspiration for your family, friends, and loved ones, so that they can get healthier.

Remember, it's not just about us; it's about everyone else we touch. The more you focus on your health — getting healthier and stronger and having more energy — the more others are going to want to do the same.

Please feel free to post your successes on Facebook or send an email; we would love to hear your story and see your results. Make sure you take before-and-after pictures. And when it gets tough, reach out to us. We are here to support you in any way we can. We have many different programs to give you the most support and take you to the next level. But at a very minimum, please feel free to send us an email, or connect with us at SmoothieShred.com.

If you have any questions or just need motivation and support, please post your questions or concerns. We will be holding regular teleseminars, webinars, and events, both online and in person. Make sure you stay on top of these updates. We would love to meet you in person!

From the bottom of my heart, thank you so much for taking the time to read this book, learn this information, and for your commitment to your health and all the others in your life whom you will inspire. Happy lifting!

Whether you are vegan or not, just remember that you are creating so much positive impact that goes *way* beyond your own muscles, leanness, and the fat you lose. Just these choices alone are going to improve your health, impact others, and help the planet. By making the decision to use this approach, you're making the world a better place. You're saving animals from suffering, improving and saving the environment from more harm, and creating more peace around the world. I want to thank you for that, too.

Next Steps

As a big thank-you for getting this far, I have some great gifts for you. Just go to my personal website, smoothiesolution.com/bookgifts.

About the Author

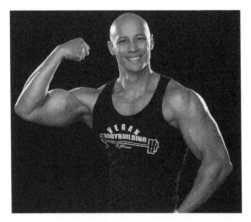

Thomas Tadlock, MS
Celebrity Trainer, Patent Holder, Author

Thomas has been recognized as one of the top trainers in the United States. His first personal training company won the *Best of Award* seven years in a row, and his second company became the largest indoor fitness Boot Camp in Orange County, California. He was MTV's 2003 Hottest Body, and is currently the host of the number-one vegan fitness and bodybuilding podcast on iTunes, the Vegan Body Revolution show, with hundreds of thousands of subscribers worldwide. He has successfully led trainings for thousands of individuals, organizations, and entrepreneurs nationwide, including professional recording artists, models, and entrepreneurs.

Thomas is a master trainer for three different fitness companies and has been featured on multiple fitness DVDs. He is highly sought-after and has worked with the top personal trainers of celebrities and professional sports teams. He holds a master's degree in exercise science and health promotion and has eight national fitness and health certifications. He is an internationally recognized trainer educator and has authored the weight-loss programs for the fitness equipment company behind the hit TV show, *The Biggest Loser*.

Thomas lives with his wife, Brooke Goldner, MD, and his two children in Austin, Texas.

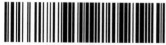

Made in the USA
San Bernardino, CA
18 February 2018